D1523483

Optimizing Bone Mass and Strength

....

Medicine and Sport Science

Vol. 51

Series Editors

J. Borms, Brussels
M. Hebbelinck, Brussels
A.P. Hills, Brisbane

Optimizing Bone Mass and Strength

The Role of Physical Activity and Nutrition during Growth

Volume Editors

Robin M. Daly, Melbourne
Moira A. Petit, Minneapolis, Minn.

24 figures, and 4 tables, 2007

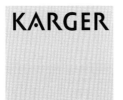

Basel · Freiburg · Paris · London · New York ·
Bangalore · Bangkok · Singapore · Tokyo · Sydney

612.75
OP7

c.

Medicine and Sport Science

Founder and Editor from 1969 to 1984: E. Jokl†, Lexington, Ky.

● ●

Robin M. Daly, PhD

Centre for Physical Activity
and Nutrition Research
School of Exercise and Nutrition Sciences
Deakin University
221 Burwood Highway
Burwood, Melbourne 3125 (Australia)

Moira A. Petit, PhD

College of Education & Human Development
School of Kinesiology
University of Minnesota
110 Cooke Hall
Minneapolis, MN 55455 (USA)

Library of Congress Cataloging-in-Publication Data

Optimizing bone mass and strength : the role of physical activity and
nutrition during growth / volume editors, Robin M. Daly, Moira A. Petit.
    p. ; cm. – (Medicine and sport science, ISSN 0254-5020 ; v. 51)
  Includes bibliographical references and index.
  ISBN-13: 978-3-8055-8275-9 (hard cover : alk. paper)
  1.   Bones–Growth. 2.   Children–Nutrition–Health aspects. 3.   Exercise
for children–Health aspects. I.   Daly, Robin M. II.   Petit, Moira A. III.
Series.
    [DNLM: 1.   Bone Development–physiology. 2.   Adolescent. 3.   Child. 4.
Exercise–physiology. 5.   Fractures, Bone–prevention & control. 6.
Nutrition Physiology. W1 ME649Q v.51 2007 / WE 200 O62 2007]
    QP88.2.O68 2007
    612.7′5–dc22

                                                          2007011221

Bibliographic Indices. This publication is listed in bibliographic services, including Current Contents® and Index Medicus.

Disclaimer. The statements, options and data contained in this publication are solely those of the individual authors and contributors and not of the publisher and the editor(s). The appearance of advertisements in the book is not a warranty, endorsement, or approval of the products or services advertised or of their effectiveness, quality or safety. The publisher and the editor(s) disclaim responsibility for any injury to persons or property resulting from any ideas, methods, instructions or products referred to in the content or advertisements.

Drug Dosage. The authors and the publisher have exerted every effort to ensure that drug selection and dosage set forth in this text are in accord with current recommendations and practice at the time of publication. However, in view of ongoing research, changes in government regulations, and the constant flow of information relating to drug therapy and drug reactions, the reader is urged to check the package insert for each drug for any change in indications and dosage and for added warnings and precautions. This is particularly important when the recommended agent is a new and/or infrequently employed drug.

All rights reserved. No part of this publication may be translated into other languages, reproduced or utilized in any form or by any means electronic or mechanical, including photocopying, recording, microcopying, or by any information storage and retrieval system, without permission in writing from the publisher.

© Copyright 2007 by S. Karger AG, P.O. Box, CH–4009 Basel (Switzerland)
www.karger.com
Printed in Switzerland on acid-free paper by Reinhardt Druck, Basel
ISSN 0254–5020
ISBN 978–3–8055–8275–9

Contents

148379

Preface

The recognition that osteoporosis is a major public health problem that is projected to escalate as our population ages has led to an ever-increasing amount of research into strategies to prevent and manage this disease. Although traditionally considered to be a disease affecting the elderly, increased recognition that osteoporosis may have its foundation early in life has stimulated substantial research interest into factors which can influence skeletal development, including both genetic and lifestyle factors. Recent advancements in bone imaging technology have also led to a rapid expansion in our understanding of the structural and biomechanical basis for changes in bone strength during both normal growth and in response to lifestyle factors such as physical activity and nutrition. With the emergence of this new information, the need for a clear, concise and comprehensive state-of-the-art account of the latest developments in this field is critically important so that health professionals, scientists and graduate students are informed of recent evidence-based knowledge on how to optimize skeletal development.

The purpose of this book is to provide a critical analysis and summary of the current state of knowledge of factors that influence the development of bone health during childhood and adolescence. The chapter by Faulkner and Bailey highlights the importance of the first two decades of life to optimize peak bone mass, with an emphasis on the rationale for adopting public health approaches to prevent this disease. The chapter by Kontulainen et al. provides new insights into the structural and biomechanical basis for changes in bone strength during growth, including a brief review of the key hormonal factors which regulate skeletal development. The chapters by Daly and by Specker and Vukovich extend this theme by examining the effects of physical activity and nutrition alone and in combination on the mass, geometry and strength of growing bone. This is followed, in the chapter by Bonjour et al., by an overview of the genetic influence on peak bone mass, and recent developments in gene-environmental interactions with regard to the skeletal responses to exercise and nutrition. The chapter by Zanker and Hind focuses on the effect of menstrual cycle disturbances and disordered eating on skeletal health in young athletes and includes recommendations for the prevention and treatment of low bone density in female athletes. The chapter by Goulding provides a thorough review of the key determinants of childhood fractures, which is followed by a concise summary by Karlsson of the latest evidence on whether exercise-induced skeletal benefits sustained during growth are maintained into old age when most fractures occur. The final chapter by Hughes et al. provides practical, real-world guidance on lifestyle strategies and guidelines, including sample programs that can be adopted by health care professionals to optimize bone health during growth.

The information in this book will benefit a range of health care professionals and scientists, including exercise specialists, pediatricians, nutritionists and dietitians, biomedical researchers and graduate students, health promotion workers and public health professionals. Specifically, for those health professionals who want a comprehensive review and critical analysis of both the existing and current literature, this book provides an excellent source of information. Public health professionals will also find this book a thought-provoking reference as it will help them understand the theoretical basis for practical exercise and nutrition guidelines to optimize bone health during growth. There is also practical information for physical educators and others wishing to add 'bone-healthy' activities to their curriculum.

Robin M. Daly, Melbourne
Moira Petit, Minneapolis

....

Contributors

Donald A. Bailey
College of Kinesiology
University of Saskatchewan
Saskatoon, Sask. (Canada)

Jean-Philippe Bonjour
Service of Bone Diseases
WHO Collaborating Center for
Osteoporosis Prevention
Department of Rehabilitation and
Geriatrics
Geneva University Hospital
Geneva (Switzerland)

Thierry Chevalley
Service of Bone Diseases
WHO Collaborating Center for
Osteoporosis Prevention
Department of Rehabilitation and
Geriatrics
Geneva University Hospital
Geneva (Switzerland)

Robin M. Daly
Centre for Physical Activity and
Nutrition Research
School of Exercise and Nutrition
Sciences
Deakin University
Melbourne (Australia)

Robert A. Faulkner
College of Kinesiology
University of Saskatchewan
Saskatoon, Sask. (Canada)

Serge Ferrari
Service of Bone Diseases
WHO Collaborating Center for
Osteoporosis Prevention
Department of Rehabilitation and
Geriatrics
Geneva University Hospital
Geneva (Switzerland)

Susan A. Novotny
School of Kinesiology
University of Minnesota
Minneapolis, Minn. (USA)

Ailsa Goulding
Department of Medical and Surgical
Sciences
University of Otago
Dunedin (New Zealand)

Karen Hind
Academic Unit of Medical Physics
University of Leeds
Leeds (UK)

Julie M. Hughes
School of Kinesiology
University of Minnesota
Minneapolis, Minn. (USA)

James D. Johnston
Department of Orthopedics
University of British Columbia
Vancouver, B.C. (Canada)

Magnus K. Karlsson
Clinical and Molecular Osteoporosis
Research Unit
Department of Clinical Sciences
Lund University
Malmö University Hospital
Malmö (Sweden)

Saija A. Kontulainen
College of Kinesiology
University of Saskatchewan
Saskatoon, Sask. (Canada)

Heather M. Macdonald
Department of Orthopedics
University of British Columbia
Vancouver, B.C. (Canada)

Moira A. Petit
School of Kinesiology
University of Minnesota
Minneapolis, Minn. (USA)

René Rizzoli
Service of Bone Diseases
WHO Collaborating Center for
Osteoporosis Prevention
Department of Rehabilitation and
Geriatrics
Geneva University Hospital
Geneva (Switzerland)

Bonny Specker
E.A. Martin Program in Human
Nutrition
South Dakota State University
Brookings, S. Dak. (USA)

Matthew Vukovich
Exercise Physiology Laboratory
South Dakota State University
Brookings, S. Dak. (USA)

Rachel J. Wetzsteon
School of Kinesiology
University of Minnesota
Minneapolis, Minn. (USA)

Cathy Zanker
Carnegie Faculty of Sport and
Education
Leeds Metropolitan University
Leeds (UK)

Daly R, Petit M (eds): Optimizing Bone Mass and Strength. The Role of Physical Activity and
Nutrition during Growth. Med Sport Sci. Basel, Karger, 2007, vol 51, pp 1–12

....

Osteoporosis: A Pediatric Concern?

Robert A. Faulkner[a], Donald A. Bailey[a,b]

[a]College of Kinesiology, University of Saskatchewan, Saskatoon, Sask., Canada;
[b]School of Human Movement Studies, University of Queensland, Brisbane, Australia

---

Abstract

Osteoporosis and related fractures are a major public health concern globally, and the
incidence and subsequent morbidity, mortality and health care costs are expected to increase
dramatically over the coming decades. Although osteoporosis was once considered (primarily) a disease of the elderly, there is now universal agreement that the condition has pediatric
antecedents. Although genetic factors play an important role in the attainment of an optimal
adult (peak) bone mass and strength, lifestyle factors such as physical activity and nutrition
are also important determinants of children's bone development. However, there is still much
research needed to identify the exact role of modifiable lifestyle factors and childhood illness
on long-term adult bone health and fracture risk. Much of our current knowledge is based on
bone mineral content and areal bone mineral density assessed by dual-energy X-ray absorptiometry; but with rapidly advancing technology, researchers will be able to more accurately
assess other indices of bone strength, such as the material and structural properties of bone,
during the growing years. Based on our current knowledge, however, it is clear that intervention strategies aimed at reducing the incidence of osteoporosis must begin in childhood or
adolescence if they are to have maximal effect.

Copyright © 2007 S. Karger AG, Basel

Osteoporosis: The Size of the Problem

Osteoporosis has often been referred to as a 'silent condition' because it
has no signs or symptoms until a fracture occurs. By definition, osteoporosis
is characterized by low bone mass and microarchitectural deterioration leading
to a reduction in bone strength with a resulting increase in the susceptibility
to fracture. It is estimated that 200 million people worldwide are affected by
osteoporosis [1], and the prevalence is continuing to increase primarily due to
the ageing of the population [2]. For instance, in the United States the prevalence
of osteoporosis is expected to increase from 10 to 12 million among individuals

over the age of 50 by 2010, and to nearly 14 million individuals by 2020 [3]. Similarly, the proportion of the Swiss population with osteoporosis is expected to increase by 8% over the next 15 years [4], and in Australia the prevalence of osteoporosis-related conditions is predicted to increase from 10% of the population currently to 13.2% by 2021 [5].

The most devastating clinical consequence of osteoporosis is fracture; it is estimated that up to 90% of all fractures can be attributed to osteoporosis [6]. Current estimates indicate that about 30–50% of women and 15–30% of men will suffer a fracture related to osteoporosis in their lifetime [7]. The most common osteoporotic fracture sites are the hip, spine and distal forearm. Hip fractures are the most serious because they require hospitalization, and are associated with significant pain, reduced morbidity, disability and excess mortality [8, 9]. It has been reported that after sustaining a hip fracture 20% of people die within the first year [10], 40% are unable to walk independently and 60% require long-term care a year later [11]. Worldwide it is estimated that there are 1.6 million hip fractures per year, and this could escalate to between 4.5 and 6.3 million by 2050 [12, 13]. Although there is considerable variation in hip fracture rates between populations, the incidence increases exponentially with age in both men and women from around the age of 60 [14]. However, the age-adjusted incidence of hip fractures in women is about twice that in men, which has been attributed to greater age-related bone loss, a higher incidence of falls, and a longer life expectancy in women [14, 15].

Vertebral fractures are also a major concern as they too are associated with substantial disability and morbidity, including decreased function, back pain, loss of height, deformity and reduced quality of life [14]. The epidemiology of vertebral fractures, however, has been more difficult to define due to the lack of a universally accepted definition for a spine fracture and the fact that many fractures do not come to clinical attention [10]. A recent review reported that the lifetime risk of a clinical vertebral fracture at age 50 years ranged from 3.1 to 15.6% in women and from 1.2 to 8.3% in men across different countries [16]. As with hip fractures, the incidence of vertebral fractures increases with age in both sexes [16], but in younger adults (<65 years) more vertebral fractures are reported in men than women which is thought to be the result of trauma sustained during previous occupational or recreational activity [15]. Furthermore, there are also data showing that following a vertebral fracture there is a two- to threefold increased risk of a subsequent fracture of a different type, and at least a fourfold increase in the risk of an additional vertebral fracture [17]. This highlights the importance of identifying strategies to prevent osteoporotic fractures in order to reduce the burden of this disease on society.

An important consequence of osteoporotic fractures is the enormous economic burden, which includes both direct (e.g. health care expenditure) and indirect (e.g. lost earnings, volunteer carers, modifications and equipment) costs. In the United States, the estimated cost per year for osteoporotic-related fractures is about USD 17.5 billion, and it is projected that in the next 10 years the cost will approach USD 45 billion per year [18]; by 2040, this could increase another three- to eightfold [19]. In Europe, the total direct costs of osteoporotic fractures have been estimated at approximately EUR 31.5 billion, which is expected to increase to EUR 76 billion in 2050 based on the expected increase in the number of elderly [20]. The total cost related to osteoporosis in Australia is estimated at USD 7.5 billion per annum, of which USD 1.9 billion are direct costs and USD 5.6 billion are indirect costs [5]. A study in Switzerland reported that osteoporotic fractures account for more hospital bed days than myocardial infarction, stroke and breast cancer [21]. Hip fractures account for a large proportion of the total costs [14]. In Canada, the annual economic implications for hip fractures was estimated at USD 650 million per year, with the average 1-year cost of care equal to USD 26,527; these costs are expected to rise to USD 2.4 billion by 2041 [22]. In addition to hip fractures, other osteoporosis-related fractures, such as the spine, wrist, ribs, pelvis and ankle, also contribute to the high human and financial costs in terms of loss of productivity related to time off work and doctor visits [23]. In summary, the prognosis for osteoporotic-related fractures and the associated potential costs to the health care system is bleak and highlights the need to identify effective prevention strategies.

A Growth and Development Issue?

Bone is a dynamic tissue that continually adapts to functional needs to produce a structure that is strong enough to prevent fractures in most activities. Childhood and adolescence is a particularly important time because the skeleton undergoes rapid change due to the processes of growth, modeling and remodeling. In both males and females, bone mass increases substantially during the first two decades reaching a plateau (referred to as peak bone mass) in the late teen or young adult years; males achieve a higher peak bone mass than females largely due to a greater skeletal size. Thereafter, bone mass remains relatively stable throughout the early to mid adult years until the onset of the naturally progressive bone loss that accompanies ageing. In women, there is accelerated bone loss around the 3–6 years of menopause, after which there is a slow continual loss in bone mineral in both men and women.

The assessment of areal bone mineral density (aBMD) by dual-energy X-ray absorptiometry (DXA), that is, the amount of bone mineral per unit area of bone, has been shown to be a strong predictor of future fracture risk accounting for up to 70% of the variance in bone strength [24]. Low aBMD in old age may be the result of accelerated bone loss during ageing, or a failure to reach an adequate bone mass during the growing years. Therefore, maximizing bone mass and strength during childhood and adolescence is recognized as an important strategy to prevent osteoporosis and fracture risk in later life.

Over 30 years ago, osteoporosis was characterized as a pediatric concern waiting to manifest itself [25]. It is now almost 20 years since the following appeal appeared in a letter to the *New England Journal of Medicine:* '… we need more information about the determinants of bone gain in childhood and peak bone mass in young adults … just as lowering blood pressure can decrease the incidence of cardiovascular events, increasing bone mass and strength is likely to decrease the incidence of osteoporotic fracture, independent of underlying pathogenic mechanisms' [26]. Despite these early concerns, the majority of research, until recently, focused on understanding the mechanisms of adult bone loss rather than bone mineral accrual during the growing years. Finally, however, there now appears to be almost universal consensus that early-life experiences are important in reducing the risk of osteoporosis in later life [27] and it is increasingly recognized that osteoporosis may indeed be a pediatric concern [28].

Peak bone mass is widely recognized as one of the best predictors of bone mineral status in older adults [29]. There is considerable evidence that bone mineral accumulation during puberty is a major determinant of peak bone mass [30]. The observation that over 25% of adult bone mineral is laid down during the 2 years surrounding the age of peak linear growth emphasizes the importance of the adolescent years in optimizing bone mineral accrual [31] (fig. 1). It is estimated that there is as much bone mineral laid down during this period as an adult will lose from 50 to 80 years of age [31, 32]. Thus, optimizing bone mineral accrual during the growing years would seem to be an essential ingredient for the prevention of osteoporosis later in life.

It should not come as a surprise that childhood and adolescence is a crucial time in terms of bone mineral accumulation. By the time growth has ceased, the skeleton should be as strong as it will ever need to be and gains in bone mineral are minimal following the cessation of growth [33, 34]. It has been estimated that 50% of the variability in bone mass in the very old can be accounted for by peak bone mass attained primarily during growth [29]. With this knowledge, it is not unreasonable to assume that fracture risk in the elderly may have childhood antecedents [35]. Although peak bone mass is largely determined by heredity, which accounts for over 50% of the individual variance [36], lifestyle factors are also involved in the multifactorial circumstances required for optimal bone mineral accrual during the growing years.

To explore the possibility of optimizing bone mineral acquisition during growth and to gain an understanding of the role that modifiable lifestyle factors

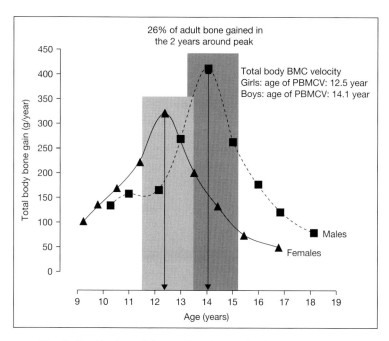

Fig. 1. Total body peak bone mineral accrual in boys and girls relative to chronological age. PBMCV = Peak bone mineral content velocity. The shaded regions represent the 2 years around PBMCV. Adapted from Bailey et al. [60].

play to promote skeletal health, it is first necessary to be cognizant of normal growth-related changes in bone mass and areal density, and the uncertainty associated with the magnitude of these changes during growth. For example, are the observed changes in aBMD an accurate reflection of change or simply a manifestation of increasing size during growth? The standard projectional methods used to measure bone density, such as photon absorption techniques (i.e. DXA), only provide a measure of aBMD in grams per square centimeter: the larger bones resulting from growth will have higher values than previously smaller bones of equal volumetric density. Thus, there has been some confusion as to the magnitude of change in aBMD during childhood and adolescence. In spite of this limitation, DXA remains the principle method of assessing skeletal status in children. Recently, the American Society of Bone and Mineral Research Pediatric Bone Initiative Group [37] recommend that, pending the development of more accurate and safe equipment, data from DXA (including bone mass and more recently estimates of bone geometry at some sites) remain the modality of choice for the near future. However, this group also recognized the need to combine traditional DXA outcomes of bone mineral content (BMC) and aBMD (where possible) with other software and bone imaging techniques that assess bone geometry and structural properties so that bone strength indices can be more accurately estimated.

Factors Affecting Bone Mineral Acquisition

Genetic endowment is the most important variable affecting skeletal growth and development; however, there also are many environmental (direct and indirect) factors that can optimize or minimize the genetic blueprint, and these factors are discussed in detail in subsequent chapters. There is a relationship between birth weight and weight in infancy and adult bone mass. Maternal smoking, diet and physical activity may all modulate bone mineral acquisition during intrauterine life [38]. Both low birth size and poor childhood growth are directly linked to hip fracture risk in later life, and maternal vitamin D insufficiency has been associated with reduced bone mineral acquisition during intrauterine and early postnatal life [39].

Childhood diseases can also affect long-term skeletal health. Juvenile idiopathic osteoporosis and osteogenesis imperfecta are examples of primary osteoporosis in children [40]. Children with growth hormone (GH) deficiency have reduced bone turnover and bone mass, and GH replacement therapy stimulates bone turnover and improves bone health in these children; however, the impact of GH deficiency during the transition to adulthood is not known [41]. Young women with anorexia nervosa are at greater risk of fracture later in life, possibly as a result of failure to achieve optimum peak bone mass or perhaps from premature bone loss associated with reduced estrogen levels [42]. Prolonged corticosteroid use in children with asthma is related to higher fracture rates in adulthood [43]. In general, chronically ill children have impaired bone mineral acquisition; thus there is a need for earlier identification and interventions in order to prevent the deleterious skeletal complications of osteoporosis that can occur in these children [44].

Although various factors during childhood influence bone growth and mineral acquisition, the most critical time for optimizing (or minimizing) skeletal development may be the peripubertal years. The main determinants of bone gain during puberty include: sex steroids (testosterone and estrogen), GH, insulin-like growth factors (by their effects on both bone and muscle mass), 1,25-dihydroxyvitamin D, calcium (calcium absorption and retention) and physical activity [30]. However, further study is needed to define the interactions among these various factors.

Nutritional quality is widely recognized as one of the most important components to optimize bone health during growth [27]; in particular, there is considerable evidence supporting the role of dietary calcium, vitamin D and protein on both bone accrual and maintenance [45]. However, the relationship between nutritional factors and bone accrual during adolescence is complicated by the large interindividual variability in the onset and duration of the maturational process in children [46]. Furthermore, there remains considerable controversy in the literature as to the accuracy of various dietary assessment methods, particularly in children. However, even allowing for disagreements on the recommended dietary intakes for calcium, there is a concern that current levels of dietary calcium are not adequate for maintenance of bone health, particularly in adolescent girls [47].

Mechanical loading through physical activity is a critical factor in optimizing bone mass and strength during growth [48]. Even small exercise-induced changes in bone mass, which are marginally detectable by DXA, may significantly improve bone strength by favorably altering bone geometry [49]. At present, however, our understanding of the effect of exercise on bone structural properties during growth is limited because there have been few studies that have used precise imaging techniques (e.g. quantitative computed tomography or MRI) to assess the cross-sectional size and shape of bone. The period of growth or pubertal development when exercise is performed may also be important; for example, the skeleton may be most responsive to mechanical loading during the prepubertal and early pubertal years [50, 51]. This conjecture is based on the hypothesis that exercise has its greatest effect on bone surfaces that are covered with a greater proportion of active osteoblasts and thus in a state of net bone formation [49]. However, whether there is a specific 'window of opportunity' during growth when exercise may have its greatest effect on bone mass and structure remains uncertain. Furthermore, even if bone mass and structure are optimized by exercise during the growing years, the clinical significance of these changes depends largely on whether the skeletal benefits are maintained in old age when fractures occur [52]. There currently remains a paucity of longitudinal data on whether there are long-term residual benefits of exercise and other lifestyle factors (e.g. nutrition) on skeletal health in old age.

Although the skeleton is amenable to a range of different lifestyle factors, genetic endowment remains a primary consideration and there is increasing information on the role of genetic factors in skeletal development and fracture risk. Parental history of fracture, particularly a family history of hip fracture, is related to increased risk of fracture independent of aBMD [53]. Recent longitudinal data do show that childhood bone size, density and strength at both the spine and femur predict values at sexual maturity, and may help predict fracture risk in old age [54]. Family and twin studies have shown that peak bone mass and bone turnover are largely regulated by genetic factors [55]. However, identifying genetic markers influencing bone development is complex because it appears that multiple genes are involved. Nevertheless, gaining an understanding of the molecular physiology of genes that influence bone metabolism will perhaps in the future enable identification of those at greatest risk and lead to the development of more specific therapeutic agents; in fact, there is some thought already that we could identify children who are genetically prone to develop low peak bone mass, and who should be targeted for osteoporosis prevention programs [54].

Issues

A primary function of the skeleton is to act in concert with the muscles to allow for controlled and effective locomotion of the body; bones must be strong to facilitate this function yet stiff and flexible to resist deformation and absorb energy by deforming so as not to fracture. Technologies have been developed to estimate various surrogates of bone strength (e.g. mineral content, skeletal architecture, geometry), but these measures alone do not provide a complete measure of whole bone strength. For example, measuring the amount of bone mineral gives no information on the geometric structural capacity of a bone. It is ultimately the whole bone structure, i.e. tissue texture or 3-dimensional tissue organization, bulk (mineral content), and morphology (dimensions, geometry), which together determine whole bone mechanical competence [56]. This is not to say that bone mineral resources are not important; indeed, bone mass remains an important component of bone strength and the relationship between mass, density and structural strength of bone and fracture holds true at all ages [27]. However, it is clear that almost all methods of assessing bone in children are influenced to some degree by growth-dependent skeletal changes [57]. Thus, as mentioned previously, interpretation of aBMD data from instruments such as DXA, where the effects of size changes are not adequately accounted for, needs to be treated with caution. There are also problems in the literature in using BMC and aBMD synonymously. BMC is size related, and although aBMD should not be, planar DXA measurements cannot fully adjust for size. Thus, the concept of a peak bone mass has been questioned and the need to assess bone strength and skeletal architecture in addition to mass has been identified [58]. If DXA aBMD values in childhood could predict aBMD values in adulthood, then it might be possible to identify children at an early age who may be predisposed to fractures later in life, and to initiate interventions at an early age; however, there is yet no clear evidence that strong bones during growth subsequently lead to a fracture-free old age [58].

As summarized by the American Society of Bone and Mineral Research Pediatric Bone Initiative [37], more research is needed on requirements for vitamins and minerals that are known to benefit bone health in children with chronic diseases. Additional research is also needed on the incidence of fractures, skeletal deformities and pain in children with chronic diseases affecting bone, and the risk factors that are the strongest correlates of fracture must also be identified.

Finally, there has never been and likely never will be a true randomized control trial examining the effects of lifestyle factors (such as nutrition and exercise) during the growing years or young adulthood on bone fragility in older age. Existing evidence is based on retrospective and prospective observation studies that are subject to systematic biases [59]. Despite these concerns, there is a tremendous consistency across trials from epidemiological studies to randomized controlled intervention studies that strongly support the important role of physical activity and lifestyle for optimizing bone development. In addition, there is considerable evidence from animal work that supports the connection of childhood skeletal development with adult bone health outcomes. This situation is similar to the knowledge base on other chronic diseases and thus, like these other conditions, further information must be gathered with as much control as possible. Interpretation of data must be objective and be based on sound biological theory and plausibility.

Conclusion

Osteoporosis is now recognized globally as a condition that has childhood antecedents. Over the past several decades, there has been tremendous advancement in our understanding of bone development during childhood and adolescence; however, much remains to be clarified through ongoing research. Genetic potential and childhood disease conditions certainly affect skeletal growth and development; however, it is clear that lifestyle factors during the growing years, particularly nutrition and physical activity, positively impact on skeletal health. Although the long-term implications of these effects on adult bone health are not yet well defined, it is prudent that public health strategies aimed at optimizing lifestyle choices be developed and implemented for children and youth.

References

1   Cooper C: Epidemiology of osteoporosis. Osteoporos Int 1999;9:S2–S8.
2   Reginster JY, Burlet N: Osteoporosis: a still increasing prevalence. Bone 2006;38:4–9.
3   National Osteoporosis Foundation: America's Bone Health: The State of Osteoporosis and Low Bone Mass in Our Nation. Washington, National Osteoporosis Foundation, 2002.
4   Schwenkglenks M, Lippuner K, Hauselmann HJ, Szucs TD: A model of osteoporosis impact in Switzerland 2000–2020. Osteoporos Int 2005;16:659–671.

5   Access Economics: Burden of Brittle Bones: Costing Osteoporosis in Australia. Canberra, Access Economics Pty Ltd, 2001.

6   Melton LJ, Chrischilles EA, Cooper C, Lane AW, Riggs BL: How many women have osteoporosis? J Bone Miner Res 1992;7:1005–1010.

7   US Department of Health and Human Services: Bone Health and Osteoporosis: A Report of the Surgeon General. Rockville, US Department of Health and Human Services, Office of the Surgeon General, 2004.

8   Keene GS, Parker MJ, Pryor GA: Mortality and morbidity after hip fractures. BMJ 1993;307: 1248–1250.

9   Autier P, Haentjens P, Bentin J, Baillon JM, Grivegnee AR, Colson MC, Boonen S: Costs induced by hip fractures: a prospective controlled study in Belgium. Osteoporos Int 2000;11:373–380.

10   Cooper C, Atkinson EJ, Jacobsen SJ, Ofallon WM, Melton LJ: Population-based study of survival after osteoporotic fractures. Am J Epidemiol 1993;137:1001–1005.

11   Magaziner J, Simonsick EM, Kashner TM, Hebel JR, Kenzora JE: Predictors of functional recovery one year following hospital discharge for hip fracture: a prospective study. J Gerontol 1990;45: M101–M107.

12   Cooper C, Campion G, Melton LJ: Hip fractures in the elderly: a world-wide projection. Osteroporos Int 1992;2:285–289.

13   Gullberg B, Johnell O, Kanis JA: World-wide projections for hip fracture. Osteoporos Int 1997;7: 407–413.

14   Cummings SR, Melton LJ: Epidemiology and outcomes of osteoporotic fractures. Lancet 2002;359: 1761–1767.

15   Sambrook P, Cooper C: Osteoporosis. Lancet 2006;367:2010–2018.

16   Johnell O, Kanis JA: Epidemiology of osteoporotic fractures. Osteoporos Int 2005;16:S3–S7.

17   Klotzbuecher CM, Ross PD, Landsman PB, Abbot TA, Berger M: Patients with prior fractures have increased risk of future fractures: a summary of the literature and statistical synthesis. J Bone Miner Res 2000;15:721–739.

18   Melton LJ: Adverse outcomes of osteoporotic fractures in the general population. J Bone Miner Res 2003;18:1139–1141.

19   Melton LJ: Epidemiology worldwide. Endocrinol Metab Clin North Am 2003;32:1–10.

20   Kanis JA: Diagnosis of osteoporosis and assessment of fracture risk. Lancet 2000;359: 1929–1936.

21   Lippuner K, von Overbeck J, Perrelet R, Bosshard H, Jaeger P: Incidence and direct medical costs of osteoporotic fractures in men and women in Switzerland. Osteoporos Int 1997;7: 414–425.

22   Wiktorowicz ME, Goeree R, Papaioannou A, Adachi JD, Papadimitropoulos E: Economic implications of hip fracture: health service use, institutional care and cost in Canada. Osteoporos Int 2001;12:271–278.

23   Center JR, Nguyen TV, Schneider D, Sambrook PN, Eisman JA: Mortality after all major types of osteoporotic fracture in men and women: an observational study. Lancet 1999;353:878–882.

24   Miller PD, Zapalowski C, Kulak CAM, Bilezikian JP: The best way to detect osteoporosis and monitor therapy. J Clin Endocrinol Metab 1999;84:1867–1871.

25   Dent CE: Problems in metabolic bone disease; in Frame B, Parfitt AM, Duncan H (eds): Clinical Aspects of Metabolic Bone Disease. Amsterdam, Exerpta Medica, 1973; pp 1–7.

26   Raisz LG: Letter to the editor. N Engl J Med 1988;795:319.

27   Heaney RP, Abrams S, Dawson-Hughes B, Looker A, Marcus R, Matkovic V, Weaver C: Peak bone mass. Osteoporos Int 2000;11:985–1009.

28   Bachrach LK: Osteoporosis and measurement of bone mass in children and adolescents. Endocrinol Metab Clin North Am 2005;34:521.

29   Hui SL, Johnston CC, Mazess RB: Bone mass in normal children and young adults. Growth 1985;49:34–43.

30   Saggese G, Baroncelli GI, Bertelloni S: Puberty and bone development. Best Pract Res Endocrinol Metab 2002;16:53–64.

31   Bailey DA, Martin AD, Mckay HA, Whiting S, Mirwald RL: Calcium accretion in girls and boys during puberty: a longitudinal analysis. J Bone Miner Res 2000;15:2245–2250.

32   Arlot ME, Sornay-Rendu E, Garnero P, Vey-Marty B, Delmas PD: Apparent pre- and post-menopausal bone loss evaluated by DXA at different skeletal sites in women: the OFELY cohort. J Bone Miner Res 1997;12:683–690.

33   Parfitt AM: The two faces of growth: benefits and risks to bone integrity. Osteoporos Int 1994;4:382–398.

34   Slemenda CW, Reister TK, Hui SL, Miller JZ, Christian JC, Johnston CC: Influences on skeletal mineralization in children and adolescents: evidence for varying effects of sexual maturation and physical activity. J Pediatr 1994;125:201–207.

35   Bailey DA, McCulloch RG: Osteoporosis: are there childhood antecedents for an adult health problem? Can J Pediatr 1992;5:130–134.

36   Krall A, Dawson-Hughes B: Heritable and life-style determinants of bone mineral density. J Bone Miner Res 1993;8:1–9.

37   Klein GL, Fitzpatrick LA, Langman CB, Beck TJ, Carpenter TO, Gilsanz V, Holm IA, Leonard MB, Specker BL: The state of pediatric bone: summary of the ASBMR pediatric bone initiative. J Bone Miner Res 2005;20:2075–2081.

38   Javaid K, Cooper C: Prenatal and childhood influences on osteoporosis. Best Pract Res Endocrinol Metab 2002;16:349–367.

39   Cooper C, Javaid K, Westlake S, Harvey N, Dennison E: Developmental origins of osteoporotic fracture: the role of maternal vitamin D insufficiency. J Nutr 2005;135:2728S–2734S.

40   van der Sluis IM, Keizer-Schrama MPFD: Osteoporosis in childhood: bone density of children in health and disease. J Pediatr Endocrinol Metab 2001;14:817–832.

41   Baroncelli GI, Bertelloni S, Sodini F, Saggese G: Acquisition of bone mass in normal individuals and in patients with growth hormone deficiency. J Pediatr Endocrinol Metab 2003;16:327–335.

42   Lucas AR, Melton LJ, Crowson CS, O'Fallon WM: Long-term fracture risk among women with anorexia nervosa: a population-based cohort study. Mayo Clin Proc 1999;74:972–977.

43   Melton LJ, Patel A, Achenbach SJ, Oberg AL, Yunginger JW: Long-term fracture risk among children with asthma: a population-based study. J Bone Miner Res 2005;20:564–570.

44   Sochett EB, Makitie O: Osteoporosis in chronically ill children. Ann Med 2005;37:286–294.

45   Bonjour PJ, Amman P, Chevalley T, Ferrari S, Rizzoli R: Nutritional aspects of bone growth; in New S, Bonjour JP (eds): Nutritional Aspects of Bone Health. Cambridge, Royal Society of Chemistry, 2003, pp 111–128.

46   Chevalley T, Rizzoli R, Hans D, Ferrari S, Bonjour JP: Interaction between calcium intake and menarcheal age on bone mass gain: an eight-year follow-up study from prepuberty to postmenarche. J Clin Endocrinol Metab 2005;90:44–51.

47   Flynn A: The role of dietary calcium in bone health. Proc Nutr Soc 2003;62:851–858.

48   Bailey DA, Faulkner RA, Mckay HA: Growth, physical activity, and bone mineral acquisition. Exerc Sport Sci Rev 1996;24:233–266.

49   Turner CH, Robling AG: Designing exercise regimens to increase bone strength. Exerc Sport Sci Rev 2003;31:45–50.

50   Petit MA, Mckay HA, MacKelvie KJ, Heinonen A, Khan KM, Beck TJ: A randomized school-based jumping intervention confers site and maturity-specific benefits on bone structural properties in girls: a hip structural analysis study. J Bone Miner Res 2002;17:363–372.

51   Lorentzon M, Mellstrom D, Ohlsson C: Association of amount of physical activity with cortical bone size and trabecular volumetric BMD in young adult men: the GOOD study. J Bone Miner Res 2005;20:1936–1943.

52   Modlesky CM, Lewis RD: Does exercise during growth have a long-term effect on bone health? Exerc Sport Sci Rev 2002;30:171–176.

53   Kanis JA, Johansson H, Oden A, Johnell O, De Laet C, Eisman JA, McCloskey EV, Mellstrom D, Melton LJ, Pols HAP, Reeve J, Silman AJ, Tenenhouse A: A family history of fracture and fracture risk: a meta-analysis. Bone 2004;35:1029–1037.

54   Loro ML, Sayre J, Roe TF, Goran MI, Kaufman FR, Gilsanz V: Early identification of children predisposed to low peak bone mass and osteoporosis later in life. J Clin Endocrinol Metab 2000;85:3908–3918.

55   Gortz B, Fassbender WJ: Genetics of osteoporosis. Orthopade 2001;30:412–417.

56 Jarvinen M, Sievanen H, Jokihaara J, Einhorn TA: Revival of bone strength: the bottom line. J Bone Miner Res 2005;20:717–720.
57 Schonau E: The development of the skeletal system in children and the influence of muscular strength. Horm Res 1998;49:27–31.
58 Schonau E: The peak bone mass concept: is it still relevant? Pediatr Nephrol 2004;19:825–831.
59 Karlsson M, Bass S, Seeman E: The evidence that exercise during growth or adulthood reduces the risk of fragility fractures is weak. Best Pract Res Clin Rheumatol 2001;15:429–450.
60 Bailey DA, McKay HA, Mirwald RL, Crocker PRE, Faulkner RA: A six-year longitudinal study of the relationship of physical activity to bone mineral accrual in growing children: the University of Saskatchewan Bone Mineral Accrual Study. J Bone Miner Res 1999;14:1672–1679.

Bob Faulkner
College of Kinesiology
University of Saskatchewan
Saskatoon, Sask., S7N 5C2 (Canada)
Tel. +1 306 966 1119, Fax +1 306 966 6464, E-Mail bob.faulkner@usask.ca

Daly R, Petit M (eds): Optimizing Bone Mass and Strength. The Role of Physical Activity and
Nutrition during Growth. Med Sport Sci. Basel, Karger, 2007, vol 51, pp 13–32

....

The Biomechanical Basis of Bone Strength Development during Growth

Saija A. Kontulainen[a], *Julie M. Hughes*[b], *Heather M. Macdonald*[c],
James D. Johnston[c]

[a]College of Kinesiology, University of Saskatchewan, Saskatoon, Sask., Canada;
[b]School of Kinesiology, University of Minnesota, Minneapolis, Minn., USA;
[c]Department of Orthopedics, University of British Columbia, Vancouver, B.C., Canada

---

Abstract

Understanding the development of the material composition and structure of bone during growth, both key determinants of bone strength, and identifying factors that regulate the development of these properties are important for developing effective lifestyle interventions to optimize peak bone strength. New imaging technologies provide the ability to measure estimates of both the material composition and structure of bone, and thus, estimates of whole bone strength. During childhood and adolescence, bone structure is altered by growth in length and width, which is associated with increases in mass, and alterations in tissue density. These processes lead to a bone with an optimal size, shape, and architecture to withstand the normal physiological loads imposed on it. Longitudinal bone growth is the result of endochondral ossification, a process that continues throughout childhood and rapidly increases during the adolescent growth spurt. Along the shaft, long bones continually grow in width, thus improving the resistance to bending forces by depositing new bone on the periosteal surface with simultaneous resorption on the endocortical surface. Sexual dimorphism in periosteal bone formation and endosteal bone resorption result in sex-specific differences in adult bone conformation. Changes in linear and periosteal growth are closely tied to changes in bone mass, with approximately one quarter of adult total body bone mineral accrued during the 2 years around the adolescent growth spurt. These structural and material changes are under mechanical regulation and influenced by the hormonal environment. Overall, bones must continually adapt their geometry and mass to withstand loads from increases in bone length, muscle mass and external forces during growth. However, the tempo, timing, and extent of such adaptations are also closely regulated by several systemic hormones.

Copyright © 2007 S. Karger AG, Basel

Failure to gain a sufficiently strong skeleton during growth may predispose an individual to bone fragility later in life. Therefore, it is important to understand both how the skeleton develops into a mechanically competent structure and the key factors that regulate skeletal development. With this information, appropriate modifiable factors can be identified and targeted for intervention to optimize the development of bone strength early in life.

The aim of this chapter is to review how bones, particularly load-bearing long bones, develop. We begin with a brief overview of the components of bone strength: bone material composition and structure. We then discuss how the commonly used bone imaging techniques, peripheral quantitative computed tomography (pQCT) and dual-energy X-ray absorptiometry (DXA), are used to estimate bone strength in the growing skeleton. We then summarize the processes of bone growth in length, size and mass, discuss how cortical and trabecular tissue densities change, and review what is known about the development of bone strength in both sexes. Finally, we discuss the mechanical and hormonal regulation of bone strength during growth.

Long Bone Strength: Material Composition and Structure

As an organ with both locomotive and supportive functions, long bones must be light for efficiency of movement, but must also consist of appropriate strength for load-bearing. Bones must be stiff and therefore able to resist deformation during load-bearing, but also flexible and able to absorb energy during loading by deforming. The functional strength of bone can then be defined as the ability of bone to serve these contradictory functions without fracturing. The ability of a bone to function effectively under a given load depends on the bone's material composition and the distribution of bone material in space (bone structure) [1].

Bone Material Composition

Bone is mainly composed of type I collagen impregnated with crystals of calcium hydroxyapatite. The relative amount of mineral embedded in the collagen matrix varies according to the function of each particular bone and determines the bone's material properties. If the mineral content of bone is greater than that needed for its normal loading environment, the bone will be overly stiff and brittle, whereas undermineralized bone will be tough but more susceptible to excessive deformation. Both situations are unfavorable and can lead to fracture. The appropriate compromise in material composition, based on the function of a particular bone, is likely selected by nature over the course of evolution. However, bone's material properties do change throughout ontogeny, with bone of younger individuals less mineralized and tougher than adult bone [1].

While the material properties of bone determine the maximum stress bone can sustain, it is ultimately the whole bone that fails, and thus, the formation of bone material into a mechanically competent structure is a major determinant of whole bone strength.

Long Bone Structure

Bone material is modeled into a three-dimensional structure designed to meet its mechanical demands. Long bones serve as levers for movement. When loaded, stresses and resultant strains are not uniform throughout a long bone, and therefore, the structure varies along the length and cross-section of each given bone. At the joint surfaces, long bones are primarily subjected to compressive loads [2]. As a result, the bone epiphyses are comprised mainly of trabecular bone. Trabecular bone is more porous and is composed of plates and struts of bone material. This type of bone favors flexibility over stiffness, is able to deform more, and is therefore appropriate for the compressive loads imposed on the ends of bone. In contrast, the slightly curved diaphyses of long bones are loaded in a combination of axial compression, bending and torsion [2] (fig. 1). To resist these forces, the diaphysis is comprised mainly of dense, stiff cortical bone. The shaft of long bones contains a hollowed marrow cavity, and excavation of the marrow cavity places mass further from the neutral axis, creating an efficient shape in which material is distributed at an optimum distance from the center of mass [2] to resist bending, torsional and compressive forces.

Measuring Long Bone Strength

Measuring Material Composition

Engineers use the elastic modulus (or Young's modulus) as a measure of the stiffness of any material. For bone, the material stiffness is largely dependent on the degree of mineralization or the density at the material level (fig. 2). Mineralization in its true sense is a physiological process whereby bone mineral is incorporated into the *existing* bone matrix. None of the currently available noninvasive imaging techniques have the spatial resolution to measure bone mineralization directly [3].

While elastic modulus cannot be measured directly with currently available imaging techniques, volumetric bone mineral density (vBMD) can be used as a surrogate of elastic modulus [4]. This tissue level density (defined as the mass of bone mineral per unit volume) reflects both the degree of mineralization

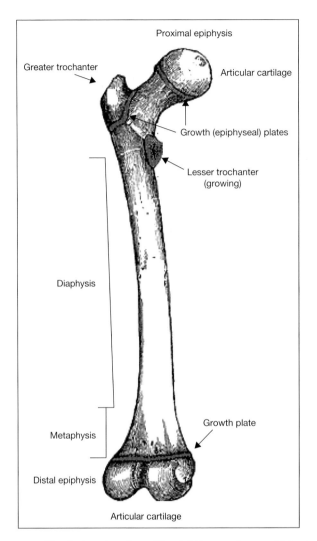

Proximal epiphysis

Greater trochanter

Articular cartilage

Growth (epiphyseal) plates

Lesser trochanter
(growing)

Diaphysis

Growth plate

Metaphysis

Distal epiphysis

Articular cartilage

Fig. 1. Anterior view of the right human femur with basic anatomy. Modified from the online edition of the 20th US edition of Gray's *Anatomy of the Human Body*, originally published in 1918.

of organic bone matrix and the porosity of the tissue [5]. Quantitative computed tomography (QCT) or pQCT allow measurement of vBMD of the whole bone cross-section, and by separating voxels into cortical and trabecular compartments, average cortical (mg/cm^3) and trabecular tissue density (mg/cm^3) can also be reported. Importantly, alterations in tissue density (vBMD) may reflect changes in mineralization and/or changes in porosity.

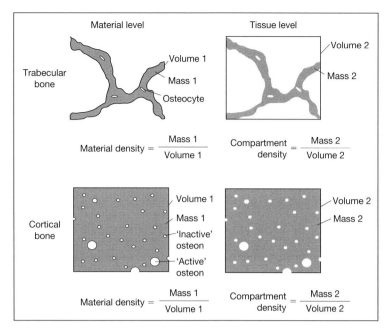

Fig. 2. Definition of density at the material and tissue level in the trabecular and cortical compartment. The mass of the mineralized bone matrix (gray) is identical at the material and tissue level (mass 1 = mass 2) but the volume differs. Material density is always higher since the volume of bone material excludes all the voids (e.g. marrow, Haversian and Volkmann canals) in bone tissue. These voids are included in the tissue density measures from (p)QCT. Modified from Rauch and Schoenau [5].

Areal bone mineral density (aBMD, g/cm^2), as measured by DXA, is not a true density, but rather a two-dimensional output representing the attenuation of photons passing through the body within the image plane only. Both bone mineral content (BMC, g) and aBMD measured by DXA have been used as surrogates of bone mineralization or strength; however, they represent some combination of those factors and are confounded by size. Nonetheless, both BMC and aBMD predict bone failure [6] and fracture risk at a population level [7]. Therefore, assessing bone mineral accrual and peak bone mass was a common goal for most pediatric bone studies prior to the development of three-dimensional imaging techniques. While these studies make an important contribution, it is important to understand what is being measured by the various imaging techniques and to recognize the inability of these techniques to independently measure structural strength and bone material properties.

Measuring Bone Structural Strength

Bone material properties alone are not adequate to represent bone strength. For example, three bones with the same bending strength can have very different density values measured by DXA or (p)QCT (fig. 3). Since the shafts of long bones are primarily loaded in bending and torsion, the strength of bone at the midshaft depends on its ability to resist tensile, compressive, and shear stresses. Indices of the structural strength of bone at the diaphysis can be gained by measuring bone dimensions (total bone area or periosteal diameter; endocortical area; cortical thickness) from imaging techniques such as (p)QCT, magnetic resonance imaging (MRI), and from software applied to DXA scans called Hip Structural Analysis (HSA).

When mathematical formulae are applied to cross-sectional images of bone at the shaft, estimates of bending and torsional strength can be calculated. The cross-sectional moment of inertia (CSMI) is essentially a measure of how effectively the cross-section resists bending or torsional loading. For bending loads, CSMI is calculated along either the x- or y-axes ($CSMI_x$, $CSMI_y$), while the polar CSMI (measured around the whole cross-section) indicates a bone's resistance to torsional loads (fig. 4). Along with CSMI, the section modulus in the x, y, or polar directions (Z_x, Z_y and Z_p, mm^3) also provides an estimate of long bone bending and torsional strength. Section modulus is derived from the CSMI divided by the maximum distance from the periosteal voxel to either the axis of bending or center of mass. Since the maximum stress that the bone diaphysis can resist before failure is inversely proportional to Z, long bone diaphyses are designed with as large a value of Z as possible [8].

Measures Combining Material and Structural Strength

As bone strength is dependent on both the material and structural properties of bone, it would be optimal to incorporate some measure of both into a strength estimate. Recently, strength estimates have been derived by 'weighting' geometric estimates of strength with density measures. The CSMI and Z assume bone mineral to be homogeneously distributed within the cortical envelope. However, the apparent density of each voxel varies due to differences in porosity and the degree of mineralization within the bone cross-section. This variation in cortical bone material properties influences bone stiffness and bending rigidity. To account for this, Z can be reported as a density-weighted Z, or strength-strain index (SSI_x, SSI_y and SSI_p, mm^3), which is derived by multiplying each voxel's area by the ratio of measured cortical density to physiologic

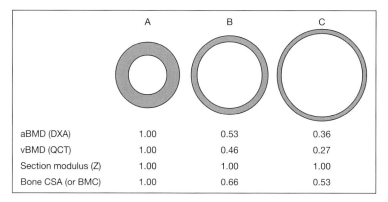

	A	B	C
aBMD (DXA)	1.00	0.53	0.36
vBMD (QCT)	1.00	0.46	0.27
Section modulus (Z)	1.00	1.00	1.00
Bone CSA (or BMC)	1.00	0.66	0.53

Fig. 3. Schematic representation of three bone cross-sections with expanding periosteal diameters (A–C) and constant section modulus. aBMD (by DXA) or vBMD (by QCT) is reduced (A–C) despite the same bone bending strength (section modulus). This is because the contribution of the bone surface to the section modulus varies exponentially with the distance from the center of mass of the cross-section; as the diameter is increased, less material is needed for the same bending stiffness. Adapted from Petit et al. [3]. CSA = Cross-sectional area.

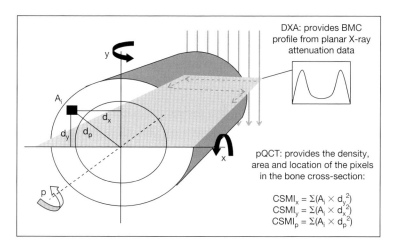

DXA: provides BMC profile from planar X-ray attenuation data

pQCT: provides the density, area and location of the pixels in the bone cross-section:

$$CSMI_x = \Sigma(A_i \times d_y^2)$$
$$CSMI_y = \Sigma(A_i \times d_x^2)$$
$$CSMI_p = \Sigma(A_i \times d_p^2)$$

Fig. 4. Schematic illustration of a tubular long-bone diaphysis and its geometric properties measured by DXA and pQCT. Whereas DXA calculates BMC from planar X-ray attenuation data, pQCT generates a three-dimensional cross-section from which geometric properties and tissue density of the bone are obtained. For example, the bending (black arrows) and torsional (gray arrow) CSMIs ($CSMI_x$, $CSMI_y$, $CSMI_p$) are calculated as the integral sum of the products of the area of each pixel (A_i) and the squared distance (d_x, d_y, d_p) to the corresponding bending (x, y) or torsion (p) axis.

bone density (1,200 mg/cm^3). The polar SSI has been shown to be closely associated with failure loads at both the radial epiphysis and diaphysis [9]. At the tibial diaphysis, both SSI and Z explain 80% of the variation in bending strength [10].

The main limitation of pQCT technology is that it is unable to measure the clinically relevant proximal femur and lumbar spine. Therefore, planar DXA measures of BMC (g) and related estimates of CSMI (cm^4) and Z (cm^3) (from HSA) provide the best currently available clinical tool to evaluate proximal femur strength development during growth. HSA is a predictive computer algorithm that incorporates the above-described mechanical engineering principles into a software-specific analysis of bone mineral data. The principle used in the HSA program is that a line of pixels perpendicular to the long bone axis in a bone mass image is a projection of the corresponding cross-section. The dimensions of this projection are used to estimate Z. Although HSA-derived femoral neck Z has been shown to be closely associated with failure load (r = 0.89) in mechanical tests [11], the assumptions related to bone shape and contribution of cortical and trabecular compartment limit the ability of HSA to reliably assess bone strength in the developing femur.

Long Bone Growth: Length, Size, Mass and Tissue Density

During growth, both bone structure and material composition are modified to produce a mechanically competent adult structure: long bones grow in length by endochondral ossification, in size by modeling (formation and/or resorption on the periosteal and endosteal surfaces), increase bone mass, and change tissue density by remodeling. In this section, we review the normal developmental pattern of these components and discuss sexual dimorphisms that occur during growth.

Bone Length

Bone growth in length occurs at the growth plate (epiphyseal plate) which is a cartilaginous template located between the epiphysis and metaphysis of long bones (fig. 1). Longitudinal bone growth is the result of chondrocyte proliferation and maturation and subsequent endochondral ossification (replacement of cartilage with bony tissue) in the epiphyseal growth plates. For bones to grow in length, newly formed cartilage is invaded by blood vessels which carry bone cells (osteoclasts and osteoblasts) that remodel the newly formed cartilage into bone tissue (ossification). This process continues throughout childhood and rapidly increases during the adolescent growth spurt until cartilage growth slows and eventually stops. The decline in growth rate is caused primarily by a decrease in the rate of chondrocyte proliferation and is accompanied by structural changes in the epiphyseal cartilage [12]. The programmed senescence seems not to be caused by hormonal or other systemic mechanisms but appears to be intrinsic to the growth plate itself [12]; perhaps because stem-like cells in the resting zone have a finite proliferative capacity. Gradual proliferative exhaustion is followed by epiphyseal fusion, an abrupt event in which the growth plate cartilage is replaced completely by bone. When growth ceases, usually in the early twenties (earlier in girls than boys), the epiphyseal plate completely ossifies so that only a thin epiphyseal line remains and the bone can no longer grow in length. Although bones stop growing in length in early adulthood, long bones continue to increase in size (cross-sectional area) throughout life to adapt to changing mechanical loads and perhaps to compensate for age-related losses in bone mass.

Bone Size and Geometry

Long bones grow in size and redistribute mass further from the neutral axes by a process called modeling. The increase in bone girth is a result of periosteal bone formation. At the long bone's outer surface, osteoblasts or lining cells in the cambium layer of the periosteum form new circumferential lamellae around the external cortical bone surface. At the same time, osteoclasts in the endosteum resorb bone on the endosteal bone surface around the medullary cavity. These two processes together increase bone size and position the cortex further away from the neutral axes, which in turn increases bone's resistance to bending. At the same time, these processes prevent the cortical shell from becoming excessively thick and also ensure that bones are not too heavy for locomotive purposes.

The timing and rate of cortical bone enlargement are related to pubertal development and sex. Cortical bone size increases at the tibial diaphysis, on average, 10% more for boys than girls across maturity groups [13] (fig. 5). This is supported by findings from iliac biopsies of healthy adolescents and young adults showing greater osteoid and osteoblast surface and osteoid volume in boys compared with girls on the periosteum [14].

The early literature described sex differences in bone size using radiographic measurements of the second metacarpal and the femur [15, 16]. These studies suggested that sex differences in bone size are established during the peripubertal growth period when periosteal apposition increases bone cross-sectional area to a greater extent in boys than girls. Radiographic comparisons of the second metacarpal showed that endosteal apposition occurs in both sexes

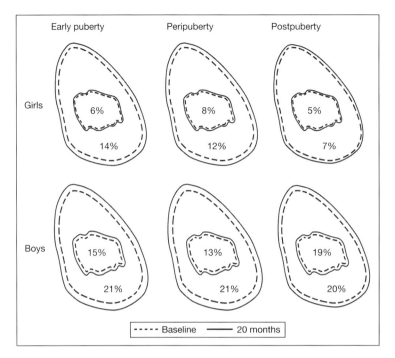

Fig. 5. Schematic illustration of cortical bone growth over 20 months at the tibial mid-diaphysis in early pubertal, peri- and postpubertal boys and girls. Numbers show the mean increase (%) in cortical and marrow cavity areas. It has to be noted that bone apposition at the periosteal (outer) and resorption at the endosteal (inner) surfaces do not occur as evenly as illustrated here. Adapted from Kontulainen et al. [13].

[15]. Since this event began earlier and was of greater magnitude in girls than boys, it was proposed that endosteal apposition in adolescent girls resulted from the pubertal estrogen surge to supply calcium for reproduction [17].

In recent years, studies have provided evidence that cortical wall thickness (estimated from DXA) increases in the femoral shaft as a result of endosteal apposition in girls [18] but not boys [19]. In contrast, recent cross-sectional comparisons of cortical bone structure by QCT [20] and MRI [21] suggested that the medullary cavity increases with advanced maturation and age in both sexes. Similarly, endocortical apposition was not evident in peri- or postpubertal girls during a 20-month follow-up [13]. The discrepancy between the earlier and more recent studies may reflect either site specificity of the phenomenon (i.e., load- vs. non-load-bearing bones) or differences in measurement techniques.

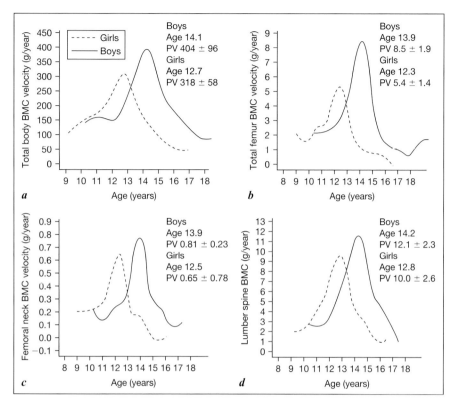

Fig. 6. Velocity curves for bone mineral accrual for the total body, proximal femur, femoral neck, and the lumbar spine for boys and girls. Note the difference in the magnitude of the bone mineral gain at peak between boys and girls, together with the timing of peak bone accrual velocities, with the girls always slightly in advance of boys. From Khan et al. [23]. PV = Peak velocity (g/year).

Bone Mass

The longitudinal University of Saskatchewan Pediatric Bone Mineral Accrual Study was the first to describe rates of bone mineral accretion, linear growth velocity, and sex differences in the timing and magnitude of bone development [22]. In this study, BMC was measured in approximately 200 children annually for 7 years. A unique aspect of these data is that researchers controlled for maturational differences that are inevitable during growth by aligning all children on a common biological maturity landmark, peak height velocity. With maturational differences between sexes controlled for, the velocity curves shown in figure 6a–d clearly illustrate a sex difference in the timing of peak bone mineral accrual [23]. For the total body, peak accrual occurred about 1.4 years earlier in girls than in boys, but was of a lesser magnitude in the girls (318 ± 58 g/year for girls versus 404 ± 96 g/year for boys). When accrual rates were compared controlling for maturational differences, boys gained significantly more bone during the 2 years around peak bone gain compared with girls and reached maturity with substantially more bone than girls [22]. For both boys and girls, more than 27% of femoral neck BMC was laid down during the 2 years around peak height velocity, and on average, 26% of adult total body bone mineral was accrued during these 2 critical years [22]. Interestingly, peak height velocity occurred ~1 year prior to the age of peak bone mineral accrual velocity in both boys and girls. This 1-year period coincides with an increase in forearm fractures in children [24]. It has been suggested that this is a time of relative skeletal fragility when linear growth is high with a 'lag' in bone mineralization. However, none of the currently available imaging techniques can accurately measure bone mineralization, thus we look to measures of cortical and trabecular tissue density to provide some insight into this important question.

Bone Tissue Density

Cortical Density

Early cross-sectional studies using QCT to assess spine or femur cortical density suggested that cortical density does not change during growth and is similar between boys and girls [25]. In recent years, however, cross-sectional and longitudinal pQCT studies have reported opposite results. Adolescent girls after Tanner stage III and adult women had 3–4% higher cortical density at the proximal radius compared with their maturity- and age-matched male counterparts [26]. These data are supported by a recent prospective study that showed a gradual increase in cortical density at the tibial shaft in pubertal girls over 2 years [27]. It has been suggested that the increase in cortical density during puberty for girls is a way of storing mineral for reproductive purposes [28]. It appears that this increased consolidation of cortical bone occurs specifically at the subcortical and midcortical regions in pubertal girls compared to boys [29].

A higher cortical density in girls could be explained by either reduced cortical porosity or an increased material density (mineralization) compared to boys. However, pQCT has insufficient spatial resolution to distinguish between these mechanisms, although evidence from cadaver studies suggests that the differences are due to tissue porosity rather than mineralization of the material [30]. Increased tissue porosity in boys may be due to higher mechanical demands (from greater body size and muscle forces) that result in increased microdamage and higher rates of intracortical remodeling [31]. Future studies are needed to confirm these findings. As mentioned previously, higher cortical density increases bone stiffness, which may provide an explanation for the lower periosteal bone formation observed in pubertal girls compared to boys [29] – due to higher cortical density, female bone may not require as large an increase in bone cross-sectional area as that required in male bone to achieve similar bone strength.

Trabecular Density

Similar to the studies describing cortical density development, there is currently disagreement in the literature as to whether there are sex differences in trabecular density development. Cross-sectional pQCT data suggest boys have *higher* trabecular density at the distal radius than girls [32]. In contrast, longitudinal data showed no sex differences in trabecular density (by QCT) at the lumbar spine, although increases were seen in both boys and girls (~18%) across puberty [33]. Discrepant findings between the axial and appendicular skeleton may reflect the more transient nature of the trabeculae within the metaphyseal region of the distal radius [32] or a difference in data acquisition, analysis and study designs (cross-sectional vs. longitudinal) [33]. Due to inadequate resolution, standard QCT measurements cannot separate trabecular number, trabecular thickness or mean material density of the trabeculae [32]. However, recent data using high-resolution pQCT to measure the distal radius suggest the sex differences may be due to greater trabecular bone volume and trabecular thickness in men, rather than increased trabecular number [34].

Overall, the limited data to date suggest that girls have higher cortical bone density, possibly due to lower remodeling rates, but lower trabecular volume and thickness than boys. Further prospective investigations are clearly needed to confirm these findings.

Bone Strength

Data from a longitudinal study with adolescent girls and young adult women showed that bone strength (as estimated with HSA-derived Z) continued to increase in late adolescence, despite no change in aBMD [35]. The magnitude of the increase in bone strength during growth is substantial. For example, when Z (measured by pQCT) at the proximal radius was compared between children (6 years of age) and adults (40 years of age), there was a difference of about 300–400% [36]. Although both sexes experienced age-related gains in bone strength, the larger bone size in boys conferred a strength advantage that was observed after Tanner stage II at the radius [36] and during prepuberty (Tanner stage I) at the tibia [37]. Similarly, at the tibial midshaft, 20-month

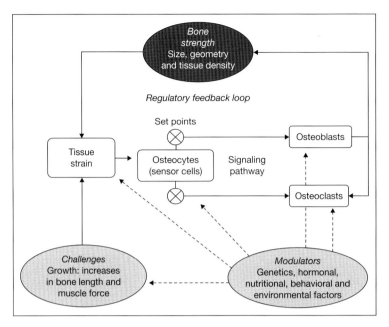

Fig. 7. A functional model of regulation of bone strength development during growth. This model is based on Frost's mechanostat theory. Modified from Rauch and Schoenau [39].

changes in Z were 14–16% greater in early pubertal, peri- and postpubertal boys compared with girls of comparable maturity status [37]. The sex difference in bone strength change mirrored the sex difference in cortical area change [37]. Although these differences may, in part, be explained by larger body size in males, females also have smaller musculature than men. Thus, lower bone strength in females may be an adaptation to smaller muscle forces and lower bending moments compared with males. This will be discussed in more detail in the following section.

Regulation of Bone Strength Development

During growth, bones must continually adapt their geometry and mass to withstand loads from increases in length and muscle mass and forces. According to Frost's [38] mechanostat theory, the mechanical competence of the skeleton is principally maintained by a mechanosensory feedback mechanism, which senses load-induced deformations (strain), and responds to maintain the skeletal rigidity through structural adaptation (fig. 7). The mechanostat model postulates that the growing skeleton regulates its strength to maintain structural integrity and to keep mechanical strains within an acceptable range [39]. During growth, the primary mechanical challenges to the mechanostat come from increases in bone length and muscle force. In addition, the theoretical mechanostat is modulated by hormones, nutrition and physical activity. These factors may affect the mechanostat via their influence on the primary challengers (longitudinal growth or muscle force), the theoretical mechanostat set point (that determines the strain magnitude at which bone tissue will react) and/or the basic multicellular unit (osteoblasts and osteoclasts) [39] (fig. 7).

Muscle Development and Bone Strength

In recent years, researchers have noted a tight relationship between changes in muscle mass and size and bone development. Muscle forces incur the largest loads on bone and thus, muscle mass or size is often used as a surrogate for the mechanical loads placed on bone. Several studies have reported a close relationship between muscle (DXA-derived total body or regional lean mass or pQCT or MRI muscle cross-sectional area) and bone development in pubertal children [40–43]. Interestingly, the relationship between muscle cross-sectional area and bone mass, size and strength in the upper limbs seems to be sex specific; upper limb muscle size is highly correlated with a change in humeral strength in males, but is much less closely related in females [44]. Furthermore, muscular development seems to have more of an effect on estimates of humeral strength than on femoral or tibial strength.

At present, it is not possible to directly measure skeletal loads (in vivo strains) that result from muscle forces. However, since muscle force scales with muscle size, muscle cross-sectional area can be used as an index of local skeletal load. However, focusing solely on muscle cross-sectional area excludes other aspects of muscle force production such as fiber type, pennation angle or neural control, which may play a role in stimulation of bone development. Researchers have used ground reaction forces of different movements or vertical jump height to represent muscle power [45]. Notably, vertical jump height, particularly in children, may be largely indicative of neuromuscular function rather than muscle power alone. Interestingly, body weight together with vertical jump performance explained the same amount of variance in bone strength as muscle cross-sectional area alone [41]. Nevertheless, muscle cross-sectional area may provide a representation of both body size and an estimation of muscle force and power.

Hormonal Factors Regulating Bone Growth

According to the original mechanostat theory, and recent modifications to it, bone strength development is modulated by genetic, nutritional and hormonal factors; however, these modulators cannot replace the direct effect of mechanical strain on the regulation of bone strength. In the following section, we briefly review the role of key hormonal factors which regulate bone growth in length, size and tissue density.

Longitudinal Bone Growth

Longitudinal bone growth is influenced directly by several systemic hormones which govern the process of endochondral ossification including: growth hormone (GH), insulin-like growth factor I (IGF-I), glucocorticoids, thyroid hormone, sex hormones, vitamin D, and leptin. These hormones are thought to regulate growth plate function either directly by acting on growth plate chondrocytes or indirectly by modulating other endocrine signals in the network [46].

Sex differences in the timing, tempo and duration of the pubertal growth spurt may be mediated by estrogen-induced stimulation of the GH/IGF-I axis. Before puberty, basal levels of the GH/IGF-I axis maintain slow and continuous bone growth [47]. Puberty is triggered by increased pulsatile secretion of gonadotropin-releasing hormone by the hypothalamus, leading to increases in serum gonadotropins and gonadal secretion of sex steroids. The increases in serum estrogen, in turn, enhance pulsatile GH secretion in both sexes, resulting in increased serum and osteoblast IGF-I concentrations.

Bone Size

The sexual dimorphism in bone size may be related to differential effects of sex steroids on the periosteal surface during development. Androgens are thought to increase cortical bone size by stimulating periosteal apposition through the androgen and estrogen receptor alpha pathways [48]. Estrogen receptor beta may mediate growth-limiting effects of estrogens in females, but does not seem to be involved in the regulation of bone size in males [48, 49]. This is consistent with the finding in growing rats that estrogen suppresses periosteal bone formation [50].

In addition to studies in rodents that suggest androgens stimulate periosteal bone formation, selective androgen receptor modulators have provided convincing evidence of androgen-induced periosteal bone formation in male rats [51]. None of these animal models are completely estrogen deficient, so it is possible that some exposure to estrogen is required to facilitate or allow androgen action on the periosteum [48]. For instance, in an aromatase-deficient boy, the anabolic action of androgens required exposure to estrogens [48].

Estrogen might also increase the mechanical sensitivity of the periosteum via estrogen receptor alpha and/or affect circulating IGF-I levels [52]. Alternatively, higher concentrations of estrogen might inhibit periosteal bone apposition and prevent the beneficial effects of loading (possibly via estrogen receptor beta) [49] on periosteal apposition.

Greater bone size in postpubertal boys compared with postpubertal girls is likely due to direct and indirect (via muscle mass and force) effects of the pubertal increase in serum testosterone since GH secretion and IGF-I production are similar or even greater in pubertal girls than in boys [47]. GH directly, and indirectly through IGF-I, stimulates osteoblast proliferation and activity, promoting bone formation. It also stimulates osteoclast differentiation and activity, promoting bone resorption. The result is an increase in the overall rate of bone remodeling, with a net effect of bone accumulation. Other hormones, such as glucocorticoids, vitamin D and leptin, may also affect bone formation at various skeletal sites but their effects on periosteal bone formation have not been well examined.

Tissue Density

Few data have directly explored the relationship between hormones and cortical or trabecular bone tissue density. It has been proposed that estrogen is responsible for the greater increase in cortical density in girls compared to boys. Specifically, the increased cyclical secretion of estrogens after menarche is thought to lead to reduced bone turnover, decreased intracortical remodeling, and less porous cortical tissue [53]. However, more research in this area is warranted.

Summary and Conclusions

During the adolescent years, long bones are rapidly growing in length and size, accruing bone mineral, and modeling to develop a structure that is light enough for locomotive activity, but strong enough to withstand loads imposed on it without fracturing. While some of these processes continue throughout life, the rate and the absolute amount of growth observed during childhood and adolescence has led to the notion that these years represent a critical time for optimizing bone health. If lifestyle factors (particularly physical activity and nutrition) are optimized, children can end adolescence with a strong adult skeleton which may potentially offset bone fragility later in life. These periods also represent a vulnerable time in which failure to properly develop a strong skeleton because of insufficient mechanical loading, hormonal insufficiency, or disease may predispose one to bone fragility and subsequent fracture in the later decades of life.

As reviewed in this chapter, novel noninvasive imaging technologies have allowed measurement of more than just bone mass or density, and have enabled researchers to better characterize normal skeletal development. While evidence suggests that longitudinal growth from the cartilaginous epiphyseal plates is under hormonal regulation, increased mechanical demands placed on bones from longitudinal growth and rapid increases in muscle development provide the impetus for bone growth in width and (re)modeling of the internal architecture to optimize bone structure and strength to adapt to changing mechanical demands.

Further investigation into the normal developmental patterns of bone and the mechanical, hormonal, and other regulators of these processes is needed. With this information, clinicians and researchers will be better able to identify deviations from normal development, and more accurately define and develop effective interventions to optimize skeletal development during the crucial prepubertal and adolescent years.

References

1   Currey JD: The many adaptations of bone. J Biomech 2003;36:1487–1495.
2   Hayes WC, Bouxsein ML: Biomechanics of cortical and trabecular bone: implications for assessment of fracture risk; in Mow VC, Hayes WC (eds): Basic Orthopaedic Biomechanics. Philadelphia, Lippincott-Raven, 1997.
3   Petit MA, Beck TJ, Kontulainen SA: Examining the developing bone: what do we measure and how do we do it? J Musculoskelet Neuronal Interact 2005;5:213–224.
4   Ferretti Jl, Capozza RF, Zanchetta JR: Mechanical validation of a tomographic (pQCT) index for noninvasive estimation of rat femur bending strength. Bone 1996;18:97–102.
5   Rauch F, Schoenau E: Changes in bone density during childhood and adolescence: an approach based on bone's biological organization. J Bone Miner Res 2001;16:597–604.
6   Manske SI, Liu-Ambrose T, de Bakker PM, Liu D, Kontulainen S, Guy P, Oxland TR, McKay HA: Femoral neck cortical geometry measured with magnetic resonance imaging is associated with proximal femur strength. Osteoporos Int 2006;17:1539–1545.
7   Johnell O, Kanis JA, Oden A, Johansson H, De Laet C, Delmas P, Eisman JA, Fujiwara S, Kroger H, Mellstrom D, Meunier PJF, Melton L Jr, O'Neill T, Pols H, Reeve J, Silman A, Tenenhouse A: Predictive value of BMD for hip and other fractures. J Bone Miner Res 2005;20:1185–1194.
8   Beer FP, Johnston ER, Dewolf JT: Mechanics of Materials, ed 2. New York, McGraw-Hill, 1992.
9   Muller ME, Webber CE, Bouxsein ML: Predicting the failure load of the distal radius. Osteoporos Int 2003;14:345–352.
10 Kontulainen S, Johnston J, Liu D, Leung C, Oxland T, McKay H: Strength indices from pQCT imaging predict up to 86% of the variation in failure load at distal and shaft sites of human tibia. J Musculoskelet Neuronal Interact, submitted.
11 Beck TJ, Ruff CB, Warden KE, Scott WW Jr, Rao GU: Predicting femoral neck strength from bone mineral data: a structural approach. Invest Radiol 1990;25:6–18.
12 Ballock RT, O'Keefe RJ: Physiology and pathophysiology of the growth plate. Birth Defects Res C Embryo Today 2003;69:123–143.
13 Kontulainen SA, Macdonald HM, Khan KM, McKay HA: Examining bone surfaces across puberty: a 20-month pQCT trial. J Bone Miner Res 2005;20:1202–1207.
14 Parfitt AM, Travers R, Rauch F, Glorieux FH: Structural and cellular changes during bone growth in healthy children. Bone 2000;27:487–494.

15   Garn SM: The Earlier Gain and Later Loss of Cortical Bone. Springfield, CC Thomas, 1970.

16   Ruff CB, Hayes WC: Cross-sectional geometry of Pecos Pueblo femora and tibiae – a biomechanical investigation. 2. Sex, age, and side differences. Am J Phys Anthropol 1983;60:383–400.

17   Jarvinen TLN, Kannus P, Sievanen H: Estrogen and bone: a reproductive and locomotive perspective. J Bone Miner Res 2003;18:1921–1931.

18   Bass S, Delmas PD, Pearce G, Hendrich E, Tabensky A, Seeman E: The differing tempo of growth in bone size, mass, and density in girls is region-specific. J Clin Invest 1999;104:795–804.

19   Bradney M, Karlsson MK, Duan Y, Stuckey S, Bass S, Seeman E: Heterogeneity in the growth of the axial and appendicular skeleton in boys: implications for the pathogenesis of bone fragility in men. J Bone Miner Res 2000;15:1871–1878.

20   Gilsanz V, Kovanlikaya A, Costin G, Roe TF, Sayre J, Kaufman F: Differential effect of gender on the sizes of the bones in the axial and appendicular skeletons. J Clin Endocrinol Metab 1997;82: 1603–1607.

21   Hogler W, Blimkie CJ, Cowell CT, Kemp AF, Briody J, Wiebe P, Farpour-Lambert N, Duncan CS, Woodhead HJ: A comparison of bone geometry and cortical density at the mid-femur between prepuberty and young adulthood using magnetic resonance imaging. Bone 2003;33:771–778.

22   Bailey DA, Maring AD, McKay HA, Whiting S, Mirwald R: Calcium accretion in girls and boys during puberty: a longitudinal analysis. J Bone Miner Res 2000;15:2245–2250.

23   Khan K, Mckay H, Kannus P, Bailey D, Wark J, Bennell K: Physical Activity and Bone Health. Champaign, Human Kinetics Publishers, 2001.

24   Bailey DA, Wedge JH, McCulloch RG, Martin AD, Benhardson SC: Epidemiology of fractures of the distal end of the radius in children as associated with growth. J Bone Joint Surg 1989;71A: 125–130.

25   Mora S, Goodman W, Loro M, Roe T, Sayre J, Gilsanz V: Age-related changes in cortical and cancellous vertebral bone density in girls: assessment with quantitative CT. AJR Am J Roentgenol 1994;162:405–409.

26   Kontulainen S, Sievanen H, Kannus P, Pasanen M, Vuori I: Effect of long-term impact-loading on mass, size, and estimated strength. J Bone Miner Res 2003;18:352–359.

27   Wang Q, Alen M, Nicholson P, Lyytikainen A, Suuriniemi M, Helkala E, Suominen H, Cheng S: Growth patterns at distal radius and tibial shaft in pubertal girls: a 2-year longitudinal study. J Bone Miner Res 2005;20:954–961.

28   Schoenau E, Neu CM, Mokov E, Wassmer G, Manz F: Influence of puberty on muscle area and cortical bone area of the forearm in boys and girls. J Clin Endocrinol Metab 2000;85: 1095–1098.

29   Kontulainen SA, Macdonald HM, McKay HA: Change in cortical bone density and its distribution differ between boys and girls during puberty. J Clin Endocrinol Metab 2006;91:2555–2561.

30   Bousson V, Bergot C, Meunier A, Bardot F, Parlier-Cuau C, Laval-Jeantet AM, Laredo JD: CT of the middiaphyseal femur: cortical bone mineral density and relation to porosity. Radiology 2000;217:179–187.

31   Pearson OM, Lieberman DE: The aging of Wolff's 'law': ontogeny and responses to mechanical loading in cortical bone. Am J Phys Anthropol 2004;(suppl 39):63–99.

32   Neu CM, Rauch G, Manz F, Schoenau E: Modeling of cross-sectional bone size, mass and geometry at the proximal radius: a study of normal bone development using peripheral quantitative computed tomography. Osteoporos Int 2001;12:538–547.

33   Loro ML, Sayre J, Roe TF, Goran MI, Kaufman FR, Gilsanz V: Early identification of children predisposed to low peak bone mass and osteoporosis later in life. J Clin Endocrinol Metab 2000;85:3908–3918.

34   Khosla S, Melton LJ 3rd, Achenbach SJ, Oberg AL, Riggs BL: Hormonal and biochemical determinants of trabecular microstructure at the ultradistal radius in women and men. J Clin Endocrinol Metab 2006;91:885–891.

35   Petit MA, Beck TJ, Lin HM, Bentley C, Legro RS, Lloyd T: Femoral bone structural geometry adapts to mechanical loading and is influenced by sex steroids: the Penn State Young Women's Health Study. Bone 2004;35:750–759.

36   Schoenau E, Neu CM, Rauch F, Manz F: The development of bone strength at the proximal radius during childhood and adolescence. J Clin Endocrinol Metab 2001;86:613–618.

37 Macdonald HM, Kontulainen SA, MacKevlie-O'Brien KJ, Petit MA, Janssen P, Khan KM, McKay HA: Maturity- and sex-related changes in tibial bone geometry, strength and muscle-bone indices during growth: a 20-month pQCT study. Bone 2005;36:1003–1011.

38 Frost HM: Bone 'mass' and the 'mechanostat': a proposal. Anat Rec 1987;219:1–9.

39 Rauch F, Schoenau E: The developing bone: slave or master of its cells and molecules? Pediatr Res 2001;50:309–314.

40 Schoenau E, Neu C, Beck B, Manz F, Rauch F: Bone mineral content per muscle cross-sectional area as an index of the functional muscle-bone unit. J Bone Miner Res 2002;17:1095–1101.

41 Macdonald H, Kontulainen S, Petit M, Janssen P, McKay H: Bone strength and its determinants in pre- and early pubertal boys and girls. Bone 2006;39:598–608.

42 Rauch F, Bailey D, Baxter-Jones A, Mirwald R, Faulkner R: The 'muscle-bone unit' during the pubertal growth spurt. Bone 2004;34:771–775.

43 Petit MA, Beck TJ, Shults J, Zemel BS, Foster B, Leonard MB: Proximal femur bone geometry is appropriately adapted to lean mass in overweight children and adolescents. Bone 2005;36: 568–576.

44 Ruff C: Growth in bone strength, body size and muscle size in a juvenile longitudinal sample. Bone 2003;33:317–329.

45 Kasabalis A, Douda H, Tokmakidis SP: Relationship between anaerobic power and jumping of selected male. Percept Mot Skills 2005;100:607–614.

46 Nilsson A, Ohlsson C, Isaksson O, Lindahl A, Isgaard J: Hormonal regulation of longitudinal bone growth. Eur J Clin Nutr 1994;48:S150–S158.

47 Riggs BL, Khosla S, Melton LJI: Sex steroids and the construction and conservation of the adult skeleton. Endocr Rev 2002;23:279–302.

48 Vanderschueren D, Venken K, Ophoff J, Bouillon R, Boonen S: Clinical review: sex steroids and the periosteum – reconsidering the roles. J Clin Endocrinol Metab 2006;91:378–382.

49 Saxon LK, Turner CH: Estrogen receptor beta: the antimechanostat. Bone 2005;36:185–192.

50 Turner RT, Backup P, Sherman PJ, Hill E, Evans GI, Spelsberg TC: Mechanism of action of estrogen on intramembranous bone formation. Endocrinology 1992;131:883–889.

51 Turner RT, Wakley GK, Hannon KS. Differential effects of androgens on cortical bone histomorphometry in gonadectomized male and female rats. J Orthop Res 1990;8:612–617.

52 Lanyon L, Armstrong V, Ong D, Zaman G, Price J: Is estrogen receptor alpha key to controlling bones' resistance to fracture? J Endocrinol 2004;182:183–191.

53 Vaananen HK, Harkonen PL: Estrogen and bone metabolism. Maturitas 1996;23 Suppl:S65–S69.

Saija A. Kontulainen
College of Kinesiology
University of Saskatchewan, 87 Campus Drive
Saskatoon, Sask., SK S7N 5B2 (Canada)
Tel. +1 306 966 1077, Fax +1 306 966 6464, E-Mail saija.kontulainen@usask.ca

Daly R, Petit M (eds): Optimizing Bone Mass and Strength. The Role of Physical Activity and
Nutrition during Growth. Med Sport Sci. Basel, Karger, 2007, vol 51, pp 33–49

····················

The Effect of Exercise on Bone Mass and Structural Geometry during Growth

Robin M. Daly

Centre for Physical Activity and Nutrition Research, School of Exercise
and Nutrition Sciences, Deakin University, Melbourne, Australia

Abstract

Regular weight-bearing exercise is widely reported to have beneficial effects on bone
mineral content and areal bone mineral density during growth, but the structural basis
underlying these changes remains uncertain. In young athletic children, participation in
high-impact sports has been shown to enhance bone formation on the periosteal and/or
endosteal surfaces of long bones at loaded skeletal sites. Participation in moderate physical
activity, recreational play or school-based exercise interventions designed to specifically
load bone have also been shown to enhance bone mineral accrual. However, few data are
available on the surface-specific effects of exercise training or general physical activity on
bone. Based on the limited data available, it would appear that the structural response of
bone to exercise during growth is maturity dependent and sex specific; prior to puberty
exercise appears to increase periosteal apposition in both sexes, whereas during or late in
puberty exercise appears to result in periosteal expansion in boys but endocortical contraction in girls. In most cases, these geometric changes lead to an increase in bone bending
strength. However, there are contrasting results as to whether the pre- or peripubertal years
are an optimal time to intervene for the greatest osteogenic response; it is likely that both
periods represent an important time for incorporating physical activity to optimize bone
health. There are also many unresolved questions as to the optimal dose of exercise (intensity, frequency, duration and rate of progression) needed to enhance bone strength in
children and adolescents. We know that weight-bearing exercise is important, and that activities should be dynamic, variable in nature, applied rapidly and intermittently, and that relatively few loading cycles are required. Although several effective interventions have been
designed for improving bone mass, further research is needed to define the specific exercise
programs or activities that will optimize bone structure and strength during growth. Perhaps
most importantly, further work is also needed to determine whether any exercise-induced
alterations in bone mass and structure during growth are maintained into old age when fractures occur.

Copyright © 2007 S. Karger AG, Basel

Osteoporosis is often considered to be a disease of the elderly because up to 60% of women and 30% of men over the age of 50 years will suffer an osteoporosis-related fracture in their lifetime [1]. As a result, there has been a great deal of research focused on identifying strategies to prevent bone loss during ageing, but the pathogenesis of osteoporosis may have its origins in childhood and adolescence. This is because the amount of bone that is gained during growth (peak bone mass) is believed to be an important determinant of future fracture risk. For instance, it has been estimated that a 10% increase in peak bone mass may delay the development of osteoporosis by 13 years [2] and could reduce fracture risk by as much as 50% [3].

While genetic factors account for a large proportion of the individual variance in bone mass and provide the template for the basic morphology of the skeleton, bone is a mechanosensitive tissue that adapts its mass, size and architecture to changes in its loading environment. There is strong evidence that growing bone is more responsive to mechanical loading (exercise) than mature bone [4]. Thus, it has been suggested that growth may be an opportune time to enhance bone mass and bone structural properties, which may increase whole bone strength and reduce the risk of fracture if maintained into later life. For this reason, there has been considerable interest in defining the appropriate mode, intensity, frequency, duration and progression of exercise, in addition to the precise timing of exercise (childhood or adolescence), necessary to optimize bone strength during growth. However, our understanding of the skeletal response to exercise has been hampered by the use of two-dimensional imaging techniques, such as dual-energy X-ray absorptiometry (DXA). This technique only provides a measure of bone mineral content (BMC) or areal bone mineral density (aBMD), and provides little information about the two important properties that determine whole bone strength: the material composition and structure of bone [5].

The development of precise noninvasive techniques, such as peripheral quantitative computed tomography (pQCT), has made it possible to measure (or obtain an *estimate* of) bone material [e.g. apparent volumetric BMD (vBMD) or 'tissue' density] and structural properties (e.g. total, cortical and medullary cross-sectional area and cortical thickness), which can then be used to provide different estimates of bone strength (bending, torsional and compressive strength). In recent years, there has been considerable interest in defining the structural basis underlying any exercise-induced increase in bone mass and strength during growth. This chapter will review the literature related to the effect of exercise on bone structural properties in children and adolescents. In addition, the evidence related to whether there is an optimal time during growth for exercise to enhance bone structural properties or tissue density will also be discussed.

The Effect of Exercise on Bone Mass, Geometry and Strength during Growth

Growth is a dynamic process in which bones continually adapt their mass, size and architecture in response to changes in mechanical load which come mainly from increased bone length and muscle forces, as well as gravitational forces associated with body weight. However, it is the muscle forces that produce the greatest loads on bone during voluntary physiologic activities. As physical activity has the potential to further increase the magnitude, rate and distribution of forces imparted to bone, it follows that bone should adapt its mass and architecture to accommodate these increased loads.

Over the past two decades, there have been many studies which have shown that exercise during growth can increase bone mass or density. However, the majority of these have relied on DXA measures of BMC and aBMD, which only provide a surrogate measure of the breaking strength of bone. Despite the widespread use of DXA and data showing that aBMD is a good predictor of whole bone strength and fracture risk, its inability to provide a precise measure of the size or cross-sectional geometry of bone, in addition to the mass distribution and internal architecture, has limited our understanding of the structural basis underlying exercise-induced increases in whole bone strength.

It is widely recognized that growing bone has the potential to adapt to increased loading through several different mechanisms (either independently or in combination): bone can be added to the periosteal surface; resorption can be reduced on the endocortical surface or bone added to increase cortical thickness; trabecular architecture can be altered (e.g. increased trabecular thickness or number), and/or bone remodeling can be slowed [6]. The clinical significance of measuring these geometric or structural changes is highlighted by data showing that changes in bone structure and internal architecture can increase bone strength with or without significant changes in aBMD [7]. This is because the resistance of bone to bending or torsional forces is related exponentially to its diameter (see chapter by Kontulainen et al., this vol., pp. 13–32, for further details) [8]. Therefore, it is likely that DXA measures alone may underestimate the effect of exercise on bone strength [7].

Effect of High-Impact Athletic Training on Bone Geometry and Strength during Growth

Cross-sectional studies of young athletes participating in weight-bearing sports that generate moderate to high impact forces (e.g. gymnastics, ballet, soccer) compared to those who engage in low-impact (e.g. walking) and non-weight-bearing activities (e.g. swimming or cycling) or less active controls have consistently reported differences in DXA-derived aBMD (or BMC) at loaded sites ranging from 5% up to 40% [9–12]. Similar site-specific gains have been reported in longitudinal studies of young athletes, particularly gymnasts [9] and ballet dancers [13]. For instance, in elite prepubertal female gymnasts followed for 12 months changes in aBMD were 30–85% greater compared to age- and pubertal-matched controls [9]. Despite these beneficial effects, only recently have studies examined the structural basis underlying the exercise-induced changes in bone mass.

A number of studies using magnetic resonance imaging (MRI) or pQCT reported large differences in bone structural and/or material properties in young athletes relative to controls. In 7- to 11-year-old female gymnasts, Dyson et al. [10] reported that total bone cross-sectional area at the distal radius (pQCT) was 11% greater in the gymnasts relative to controls, despite the gymnasts being shorter. Although this difference was not significant, the finding that trabecular and cortical vBMD were significantly greater (15–27%) in the gymnasts suggests that exercise increased the mass of bone 'inside' the periosteal envelope – this could be due to either thicker trabeculae or endosteal apposition (or reduced endosteal resorption). In a similar cross-sectional study of prepubertal male and female gymnasts, total and cortical area and the stress-strain index (an estimate of the bending and torsional strength of long bones) at the mid radius were significantly greater in the gymnasts compared to controls, but no differences were detected for cortical vBMD [14]. In contrast, a beneficial effect of gymnastics training was observed for total and/or trabecular vBMD (but not bone size) at distal skeletal sites (distal radius and tibia). In a prospective study of elite prepubertal female gymnasts, it has been reported that there was a greater increase in DXA-derived vBMD at the lumbar spine and mid-femoral shaft in gymnasts relative to controls, which was attributed to changes at the endocortical and not periosteal surfaces [9].

In high-level female adolescent athletes (distance runners), studies using a combination of DXA and MRI have reported that mid femur or distal tibia cortical area, cross-sectional moment of inertia (CSMI; an estimate of the bending and torsional strength of bone) and the bone strength index (BSI; which combines bone mineral and its distribution to measure resistance to bending) were greater compared with swimmers, cyclists and/or non-active controls [15, 16]. In these adolescent athletes, however, there appeared to be no effect of loading on total bone area (periosteal apposition). Swimmers, cyclists [15] and controls [16] had larger medullary cavities indicating increased endosteal resorption relative to the runners. Interestingly, cortical vBMD was only greater at the distal tibia (a site containing predominantly trabecular bone) in female athletes relative to controls [16]. Consistent with these findings, there is evidence that adult male and female athletes who commence training late in puberty have greater trabecular vBMD at distal skeletal sites (radius and tibia) without corresponding changes in periosteal bone area [17, 18], although in elite young adult male and female triple jumpers total bone area was 6% greater relative to controls [18].

An important limitation of cross-sectional studies involving young athletes is that they are often confounded by selection bias, that is, children who are stronger are more likely to participate and be successful in sport. To overcome this issue, several studies have compared bone structural differences between the playing and nonplaying arms of young tennis and squash players, which controls for the confounding effects of genetic, hormonal and dietary factors. In one study of former male tennis players (aged 30 ± 5 years) who started training during childhood, exercise resulted in increased total bone and medullary area (periosteal and endocortical expansion) at the proximal humerus and mid radius as measured by pQCT (fig. 1). At the mid and distal humerus, there was an increase in total bone area (periosteal expansion), but no effect on medullary area which resulted in a marked increase in cortical area and thickness [19]. There was no significant effect of exercise on cortical or trabecular vBMD at any site. Similar results were found in a study of young adult female tennis players (aged 26 ± 8 years) who commenced training at 10.5 ± 2.2 years, with the exception that exercise enhanced trabecular vBMD at the distal radius (fig. 1) [20].

In addition to assessing the effect of loading during growth on bone structural properties, a number of unilateral studies have also examined whether there is a maturity-dependent surface-specific response to loading. It has been proposed that exercise preferentially results in an increase in bone mass or altered geometry at the surfaces already undergoing rapid bone formation due to normal growth [21]. Based on this hypothesis, exercise during the prepubertal years should result in increased periosteal but not endocortical apposition. At puberty, exercise should primarily add bone to the periosteal surface in both boys and girls, whereas from late puberty to early adulthood the predominant effect of exercise should be periosteal apposition in boys and endocortical apposition in girls. This is because testosterone secretion in males results in continued periosteal apposition whereas estrogen inhibits periosteal apposition but stimulates the acquisition of bone on the endocortical surface [22].

In a cross-sectional study using MRI to compare the side-to-side differences in bone geometry of the arms of pre-, peri- and postpubertal female tennis players, Bass et al. [23] reported that exercise prior to puberty was associated with an increase in bone size (periosteal apposition) and bending strength, whereas the predominant effect after puberty was endocortical apposition with little additional benefit to the bone's resistance to bending (fig. 2). Most of the exercise-induced bone structural changes in the girls appeared to occur during the

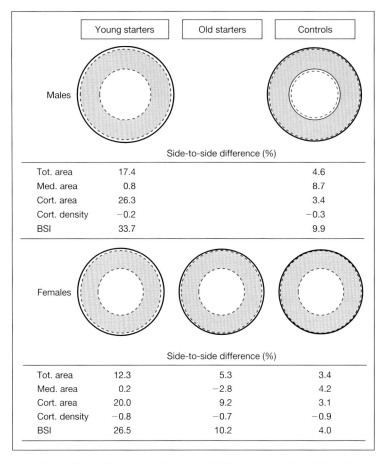

Fig. 1. Mean side-to-side differences (%) in humeral mid shaft total bone area (Tot. area), medullary cavity area (Med. area), cortical area (Cort. area), cortical density (Cort. density) and BSI (density-weighted polar section modulus) between the playing and nonplaying arm of male [19] and female [20] tennis players and controls. For each illustration, the dotted line represents the nonplaying arm and the continuous line the playing arm. Adapted from Kontulainen et al. [20].

prepubertal years. Consistent with these results, Haapasalo et al. [24] reported that the side-to-side differences in cortical thickness, but not bone size (width), were greater in female tennis players who had started training after puberty compared to matched controls. Together, these findings support the notion that exercise may enhance bone formation on the periosteal surface during the prepubertal years, with a potential effect on the endocortical surface during the postpubertal years. These findings are consistent with the hypothesis that rising estrogen

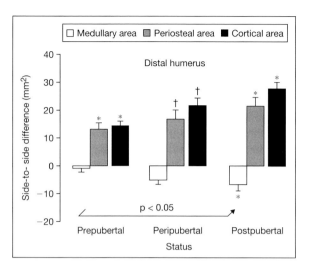

Fig. 2. Mean (± SE) side-to-side differences in periosteal, medullary and cortical bone area at the distal humerus between the playing and nonplaying arms of pre-, peri- and postpubertal female tennis players. The change in cortical area caused by loading during the pre- and peripubertal period was primarily the result of greater periosteal expansion, whereas loading during the postpubertal years resulted primarily in medullary contraction (endosteal apposition). *p < 0.001, †p < 0.01 versus nonplaying arm. Adapted from Bass et al. [23].

levels may lower the bone (re)modeling threshold on the endocortical surface, and thereby sensitize bone next to marrow to the effect of loading late in puberty [25]. However, there are also data which have shown that playing tennis has no effect on the endocortical surface in women who began playing either before or after menarche [20], and that the surface-specific response to loading may vary along the length of bone [19, 23, 24]. Thus, further research is needed before definitive conclusions can be made with respect to the optimal time during growth when exercise may enhance bone structural properties.

In summary, the results from cross-sectional and unilateral studies of athletes involved in high-impact sports indicate that the shafts of long bones, which are typically subjected to bending and torsional forces from muscle pull, undergo geometric adaptations in response to increased loading. The specific geometric adaptation appears to vary according to gender and the stage of maturation, and likely differs depending on the type of loading induced. Limited data to date suggest that increased loading during the pre- and peripubertal years in both girls and boys appears to result mainly in increased periosteal apposition whereas late in puberty the predominant response appears to be periosteal apposition in boys and endocortical apposition in girls. In contrast, at more distal skeletal sites containing predominantly trabecular bone, which are subjected to axial and compressive loads, exercise appears to result in an increase in tissue density rather than bone size perhaps to more efficiently dissipate the loads from the joint surface evenly up into the bone [14].

Effect of Recreational and Leisure Activity on Bone Geometry and Strength during Growth

There are currently few data which explore the effectiveness of regular physical activity and recreational play on bone geometry and structural strength in children and adolescents. Several studies have, however, explored the influence of recreational activity on bone mass or aBMD. In an earlier DXA-based study of healthy children aged 5–14 years, Slemenda et al. [26] reported that total hours of weight-bearing physical activity were significantly associated with aBMD at the radius and proximal femur. The authors concluded that children with physical activity levels one standard deviation above the mean (2.7 h per day) were likely to emerge from adolescence with 5–10% greater bone mass. In a subsequent 3-year observational study by the same group, they reported a 4–7% greater increase in femur aBMD for prepubertal children in the highest compared to lower quartile of physical activity [27]. Interestingly, there was no relationship between physical activity and change in aBMD in peripubertal girls (Tanner stages II–IV). The strongest evidence for a beneficial effect of everyday physical activity on bone mineral accrual comes from a 7-year longitudinal study in Canadian children. In 53 girls and 60 boys with longitudinal data spanning the adolescent years, Bailey et al. [28] reported that children in the highest quartile of physical activity accrued more bone during the 2 years around peak bone mineral accrual, and had greater BMC (femoral neck 7–9%; total body 11–16%) than those in the lowest quartile of physical activity 1 year after peak bone mineral accrual (fig. 3). Using the DXA hip structural analysis program, they reported in a subsequent study that physical activity was a significant positive independent predictor of bone cross-sectional area and section modulus (a measure of bending strength) of the narrow region of the femoral neck [29]. While the strength of these data lies in the longitudinal nature of the study and the ability to align children according to a similar maturational landmark (peak height velocity), these results must also be considered in light of the small number of children (n = 13–17) classified into the highest and lowest quartile of physical activity; the potential for sampling bias (more active children may be bigger and stronger and thus more likely to continue playing sport than less active children), and the limitations of using two-dimensional DXA output to calculate three-dimensional strength indices.

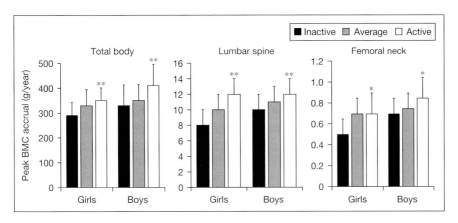

Fig. 3. Total body, lumbar spine and femoral neck peak bone mineral accrual velocity of girls and boys classified into one of three physical activity groups: inactive (lowest quartile), average (between the lowest and highest quartile) and active (highest quartile). *p < 0.05, **p < 0.001 compared to inactive. Adapted from Bailey et al. [28].

In one of the few studies to have used pQCT to examine the effects of regular physical activity on bone tissue density and structural properties, Wang et al. [30] reported that prepubertal girls with higher leisure time physical activity levels had significantly greater tibial shaft cortical vBMD and cortical thickness, but not total bone size compared with girls in the low physical activity group; DXA BMC and aBMD measures were also greater in the more active girls. In contrast, no differences were detected for tibial vBMD or geometry in peripubertal girls (Tanner stage II). Interestingly, bone size was greater in prepubertal girls who participated in more high-impact (weight-bearing) compared to low-impact activities. Consistent with these findings, a cross-sectional study of prepubertal boys and girls aged 4–7 years reported that children in the highest tertile of physical activity (>42 min per day of vigorous activity) had 7–12% higher proximal femur bone cross-sectional area and section modulus (DXA hip structural analysis) than those in the lowest tertile of vigorous activity (<30 min per day) [31].

While the findings from these studies provide some evidence that everyday regular physical activity may enhance the structural strength of bones during growth, it is important to recognize that most of these studies relied on an assessment of physical activity through a questionnaire. Given the inherent errors typically associated with trying to accurately quantify physical activity levels from questionnaires, especially in children, longitudinal exercise intervention trials are needed to quantify the effect of exercise type, frequency, duration and intensity on the material and structural properties of bone during growth.

Effect of School-Based Exercise Interventions on Bone Geometry and Strength

In the past decade, there has been an increasing number of intervention studies examining the effects of exercise on changes in BMC and aBMD assessed by DXA in normally active healthy school-aged children and adolescents. Most of these studies implemented programs consisting of weight-bearing exercises that involved either extra physical education classes or were additional to normal physical education and implemented during or after school hours for 10–45 min per session, 2–5 times per week [32–43]. The results from these studies, which varied in duration (8–24 months) and design (randomized versus nonrandomized), generally found that exercise led to relatively modest improvements in BMC and aBMD ranging from 1 to 5% according to the skeletal site. However, a few studies failed to detect a beneficial effect of exercise on bone mineral accrual [44, 45]. These contrasting results could be explained by a number of factors, including differences in the exercise programs (duration, frequency, mode and rate of progression) and the background loading history and maturity status of individuals. It is also plausible that the positive effects of exercise on bone where underestimated because most of these studies did not assess changes in bone structure or geometry which, as indicated, can influence whole bone strength independent of changes in aBMD [7].

In one of the first studies to have examined the structural basis of any increase in aBMD associated with a moderate exercise intervention in normoactive children, Bradney et al. [34] reported that the greater increase in femoral mid shaft aBMD (derived from total body DXA scans) in prepubertal boys who participated in an 8-month non-progressive school-based exercise program (30 min of weight-bearing activity 3 times per week) was due to less endocortical resorption and not greater periosteal expansion compared to matched controls. They also observed a greater exercise-induced increase in mid femur vBMD, but there was no effect of exercise on estimates of bone strength (CSMI or section modulus). This could be explained by the lack of an effect of exercise on periosteal width; a small amount of bone deposited on the periosteal surface can confer large changes in CSMI because it is proportional to the fourth power of the radius [46].

In contrast to these findings, the results from a 7-month study in prepubertal and early pubertal girls randomized to a progressive jumping exercise program (10 min per day, 3 times per week) or control group revealed that there was no additional effect of exercise on hip bone structural properties (estimated from DXA) in prepubertal girls. In the early pubertal exercise group however, there was a greater increase in femoral neck and intertrochanteric aBMD due largely to greater apposition (or less resorption) on the endosteal surface [6]. Despite the lack of an exercise effect on the periosteal surface, the structural changes on the endosteal surface of the femoral neck led to a small but significant improvement (4%) in section modulus relative to controls. These findings not only indicate that exercise during puberty in girls can enhance bone structural properties (at the endosteal surface), but also that bone may be more responsive to loading during the peri- compared to prepubertal period. There is a sound physiological basis to support this hypothesis: the peripubertal period corresponds to a time around peak bone mineral accrual when growth hormone, insulin-like growth factor I and sex steroid levels increase and enhance bone growth and turnover through osteoblastic stimulation. However, the lack of an effect of exercise in the prepubertal children in this study could be partly related to differences in the number of prepubertal girls that progressed to Tanner stage II in the control (61%) relative to the intervention group (41%). Interestingly, in pre- and early-mid pubertal boys who completed the same school-based exercise intervention over 20 months, exercise led to a trend towards greater expansion on both the periosteal (2.6%) and endosteal surfaces (2.7%) of the femoral neck relative to controls, which resulted in a 7.5–12.4% greater increase in bone strength (section modulus and CSMI) [40]. In this study however, the data for pre- and early-mid pubertal boys were pooled and thus it is not known whether there was a maturity-dependent response to loading. Furthermore, as with the same intervention conducted in girls [6, 38], the maturational progression of the boys was not similar between the intervention and control groups, and thus it is difficult to determine whether the benefits were largely due to growth-related differences or the exercise intervention.

While further work is still needed to determine whether there is a specific 'window of opportunity' during growth when exercise may enhance bone mass, the finding that exercise during growth can enhance bone structural properties is supported by the results from several other exercise intervention studies in prepubertal and/or early pubertal boys and girls. Several of these studies have reported greater gains in DXA-derived bone area at the femoral neck [32, 35] or lumbar spine following exercise training [41, 42]. However, these findings are not consistent. For instance, a recent study in pre- and peripubertal boys and girls reported no significant effect of 10 jumps 3 times per day over 8 months on DXA-derived hip bone structural parameters, despite greater exercise-induced gains in BMC at the proximal femur [47]. Due to the small sample size in this study however, it is likely they were underpowered to detect any bone structural changes that may have occurred.

While DXA-based intervention studies that have estimated the effect of exercise on bone structure and geometry have contributed to our understanding of the structural basis underlying changes in aBMD during growth, the results must be interpreted cautiously given the inherent methodological limitations, assumptions and errors associated with using a two-dimensional technique to estimate the geometry of a three-dimensional structure, particularly in growing children. Thus, it is important that we progress to more advanced imaging techniques [e.g. (p)QCT or MRI] that can provide an accurate view of the cross-sectional size and shape of bone. To date, there have only been three published exercise intervention studies that have used pQCT to examine the effects of exercise on bone structural and material properties in pre- and peripubertal children. In a 9-month jumping intervention (2 sessions per week) involving pre- and postmenarcheal girls, Heinonen et al. [36] reported no effect of exercise on cortical vBMD, cross-sectional area or BSI at the tibial mid shaft in either group of girls. There was, however, a positive effect of exercise on DXA BMC at the lumbar spine and femoral neck in the premenarcheal girls. Similar to these results, a 12-week intervention involving 54 pre-, peri- and postpubertal children randomized to either a jumping program (25 jumps per day off a 45-cm box, 5 days per week) or control group reported no effect of exercise on distal tibia (4% and 20% sites) periosteal or endosteal circumference, despite a greater increase in DXA leg BMC in the jumpers [48]. Interestingly, in this study they reported that jumping was associated with greater trabecular bone area and lower total and trabecular vBMD at the 4% distal tibia in the peripubertal girls. This suggests that loading increased trabecular area and endosteal resorption during puberty. Unfortunately, in both these studies the sample size was relatively small and thus it is also likely they had insufficient power to detect any significant beneficial effects of exercise on bone structural parameters.

In a unique 12-month randomized study in preschool children aged 3–5 years, Specker and Binkley [49] reported that children who participated in a gross motor activity program (30 min per day, 5 days per week) had greater periosteal and endosteal circumferences at the 20% distal tibia than children who engaged in a fine motor activity program. They also observed a significant interaction between calcium supplementation and physical activity for both cortical thickness and cortical area: in children receiving placebo, cortical thickness and area were smaller with gross motor activity compared with fine motor activity, but for children receiving calcium, cortical thickness and area were larger with gross motor activity [49]. While these findings indicate that exercise early in life may enhance bone structural properties, particularly in the presence of increased dietary calcium intakes, further studies are needed to validate these results because of difficulties associated with movement during the pQCT scans in a large proportion (51%) of the young children in this study.

In summary, it is clear from the limited intervention studies available that regular weight-bearing exercise can have beneficial effects on bone mineral accrual at loaded sites, but the structural basis underlying these changes remains uncertain. This is likely to be due to a number of factors, including the short duration of many intervention trials; the use of different techniques to assess bone geometry (e.g. DXA, MRI, pQCT); differences in the exercise protocols used, and the marked variability between studies for exercise compliance. Furthermore, additional research is needed before we can define the precise structural mechanisms underlying changes in bone strength in response to exercise in boys and girls. Further work is also needed to determine whether there is a specific 'window of opportunity' during growth when exercise may lead to the greatest increase in bone mass or structure, although there is sound evidence that the pre- and early-mid pubertal years are both important periods to enhance bone strength.

Whether there is an optimal dose of exercise required to enhance bone structural properties during growth also remains uncertain. We know that moderate- to high-impact weight-bearing exercise is important, and activities should be variable in nature (e.g. multidirectional) and applied rapidly and intermittently, and that relatively few loading cycles are necessary. However, the current evidence does not lend itself to the development of a specific training program that will enhance bone mineral accrual and structural strength during growth. This is because most school-based intervention trials incorporated a range of different weight-bearing activities, such as running, jumping, hopping, skipping, dancing, gymnastics activities, ball sports and weight lifting [32–43]. Further long-term studies are needed to examine the dose-response relationship between exercise and bone strength, which should include an assessment of the relative mechanical loads associated with different exercise activities in pre-, peri-, and postpubertal boys and girls.

Summary and Conclusion

There is compelling evidence that children and adolescents involved in regular moderate- to high-impact weight-bearing activities have higher aBMD and greater bone strength at loaded sites due to either periosteal and/or endosteal apposition (or reduced endosteal resorption) than those involved in non-weight-bearing sports or less active controls. Participation in regular physical activity/recreational play or school-based exercise interventions incorporating specific bone-loading activities can also enhance bone mineral accrual, but the structural basis underlying these changes remains uncertain. From the limited data available, it would appear that the structural response of long bones to exercise during growth is maturity dependent and sex specific; prior to puberty exercise appears to increase periosteal apposition in both boys and girls, whereas during or late in puberty exercise appears to result in periosteal expansion in boys but endocortical contraction in girls. At distal skeletal sites containing predominantly trabecular bone, exercise appears to result in an increase in tissue density (perhaps due to an increase in trabecular thickness or endosteal apposition) rather than size (periosteal apposition). However, further rigorous randomized intervention trials in which children are appropriately matched in terms of age, gender, race, anthropometric and maturity characteristics, and if possible, previous physical activity history and exercise training loads are required to determine the structural basis underlying any increase in bone strength produced by exercise during growth.

Whether there is a specific 'window of opportunity' during growth when the skeleton may be most responsive to exercise is also unknown. Despite sound evidence that exercise is more effective during the pre- compared to postmenarcheal years in girls, it is still uncertain whether the pre- or peripubertal years are best for boys and girls; it is likely that both periods represent an important time to enhance the structural strength of bone but further research is needed. There are also many unresolved questions as to how much, how often, what magnitude or how long children need to exercise to enhance bone strength during growth. Nevertheless, some guidelines can be made based on existing evidence (see chapter by Hughes et al., this vol., pp. 137–158). It is clear that weight-bearing exercise is important, and more specifically, activities that are dynamic, variable in nature, applied rapidly and intermittently with relatively few loading cycles all appear to be effective for enhancing bone formation. Despite this, there is still a lack of evidence regarding the most effective program to optimize bone strength during growth. Finally, and perhaps more importantly, further research is needed to determine whether any exercise-induced alterations sustained during growth are maintained into old age when the risk of fragility fractures increases exponentially (refer to chapter by Karlsson, this vol., pp. 121–136 for further details).

References

1   US Department of Health and Human Services: Bone Health and Osteoporosis: A Report of the Surgeon General. Rockville, US Department of Health and Human Services, Office of the Surgeon General, 2004.
2   Hernandez CJ, Beaupre GS, Carter DR: A theoretical analysis of the relative influences of peak BMD, age-related bone loss and menopause on the development of osteoporosis. Osteoporos Int 2003;14:843–847.
3   Cummings SR, Black DM, Nevitt MC, Browner W, Cauley J, Ensrud K, Genant HK, Palermo L, Scott J, Vogt TM: Bone density at various sites for prediction of hip fractures. The Study of Osteoporotic Fractures Research Group. Lancet 1993;341:72–75.
4   Forwood MR, Burr DB: Physical activity and bone mass: exercises in futility? Bone Miner 1993;21:89–112.
5   Seeman E: From density to structure: growing up and growing old on the surfaces of bone. J Bone Miner Res 1997;12:1–13.

6   Petit MA, McKay HA, MacKelvie KJ, Heinonen A, Khan KM, Beck TJ: A randomized school-based jumping intervention confers site and maturity-specific benefits on bone structural properties in girls: a hip structural analysis study. J Bone Miner Res 2002;17:363–372.

7   Jarvinen TL, Kannus P, Sievanen H: Have the DXA-based exercise studies seriously underestimated the effects of mechanical loading on bone? J Bone Miner Res 1999;14:1634–1635.

8   Orwoll ES: Toward an expanded understanding of the role of the periosteum in skeletal health. J Bone Miner Res 2003;18:949–954.

9   Bass S, Pearce G, Bradney M, Hendrich E, Delmas PD, Harding A, Seeman E: Exercise before puberty may confer residual benefits in bone density in adulthood: studies in active prepubertal and retired female gymnasts. J Bone Miner Res 1998;13:500–507.

10 Dyson K, Blimkie CJ, Davison KS, Webber CE, Adachi JD: Gymnastic training and bone density in pre-adolescent females. Med Sci Sports Exerc 1997;29:443–450.

11 Kannus P, Haapasalo H, Sankelo M, Sievanen H, Pasanen M, Heinonen A, Oja P, Vuori I: Effect of starting age of physical activity on bone mass in the dominant arm of tennis and squash players. Ann Intern Med 1995;123:27–31.

12 Young N, Formica C, Szmukler G, Seeman E: Bone density at weight-bearing and nonweight-bearing sites in ballet dancers: the effects of exercise, hypogonadism, and body weight. J Clin Endocrinol Metab 1994;78:449–454.

13 Matthews BL, Bennell KL, McKay HA, Khan KM, Baxter-Jones AD, Mirwald RL, Wark JD: Dancing for bone health: a 3-year longitudinal study of bone mineral accrual across puberty in female non-elite dancers and controls. Osteoporos Int 2006;17:1043–1054.

14 Ward KA, Roberts SA, Adams JE, Mughal MZ: Bone geometry and density in the skeleton of pre-pubertal gymnasts and school children. Bone 2005;36:1012–1018.

15 Duncan CS, Blimkie CJ, Kemp A, Higgs W, Cowell CT, Woodhead H, Briody JN, Howman-Giles R: Mid-femur geometry and biomechanical properties in 15- to 18-yr-old female athletes. Med Sci Sports Exerc 2002;34:673–681.

16 Greene DA, Naughton GA, Briody JN, Kemp A, Woodhead H, Corrigan L: Bone strength index in adolescent girls: does physical activity make a difference? Br J Sports Med 2005;39:622–627.

17 Ashizawa N, Nonaka K, Michikami S, Mizuki T, Amagai H, Tokuyama K, Suzuki M: Tomographical description of tennis-loaded radius: reciprocal relation between bone size and volumetric BMD. J Appl Physiol 1999;86:1347–1351.

18 Heinonen A, Sievanen H, Kyrolainen H, Perttunen J, Kannus P: Mineral mass, size, and estimated mechanical strength of triple jumpers' lower limb. Bone 2001;29:279–285.

19 Haapasalo H, Kontulainen S, Sievanen H, Kannus P, Jarvinen M, Vuori I: Exercise-induced bone gain is due to enlargement in bone size without a change in volumetric bone density: a peripheral quantitative computed tomography study of the upper arms of male tennis players. Bone 2000;27: 351–357.

20 Kontulainen S, Sievanen H, Kannus P, Pasanen M, Vuori I: Effect of long-term impact-loading on mass, size, and estimated strength of humerus and radius of female racquet-sports players: a peripheral quantitative computed tomography study between young and old starters and controls. J Bone Miner Res 2003;18:352–359.

21 Ruff CB, Walker A, Trinkaus E: Postcranial robusticity in Homo. 3. Ontogeny. Am J Phys Anthropol 1994;93:35–54.

22 Seeman E: Clinical review 137: sexual dimorphism in skeletal size, density, and strength. J Clin Endocrinol Metab 2001;86:4576–4584.

23 Bass SL, Saxon L, Daly RM, Turner CH, Robling AG, Seeman E, Stuckey S: The effect of mechanical loading on the size and shape of bone in pre-, peri-, and postpubertal girls: a study in tennis players. J Bone Miner Res 2002;17:2274–2280.

24 Haapasalo H, Sievanen H, Kannus P, Heinonen A, Oja P, Vuori I: Dimensions and estimated mechanical characteristics of the humerus after long-term tennis loading. J Bone Miner Res 1996;11:864–872.

25 Frost HM: On our age-related bone loss: insights from a new paradigm. J Bone Miner Res 1997;12:1539–1546.

26 Slemenda CW, Miller JZ, Hui SL, Reister TK, Johnston CC Jr: Role of physical activity in the development of skeletal mass in children. J Bone Miner Res 1991;6:1227–1233.

---

27 Slemenda CW, Reister TK, Hui SL, Miller JZ, Christian JC, Johnston CC: Influences of skeletal mineralization in children and adolescents: evidence for varying effects of sexual maturation and physical activity. J Pediatr 1994;125:201–207.

28 Bailey DA, McKay HA, Mirwald RL, Crocker PR, Faulkner RA: A six-year longitudinal study of the relationship of physical activity to bone mineral accrual in growing children: the university of Saskatchewan bone mineral accrual study. J Bone Miner Res 1999;14:1672–1679.

29 Forwood MR, Baxter-Jones AD, Beck TJ, Mirwald RL, Howard A, Bailey DA: Physical activity and strength of the femoral neck during the adolescent growth spurt: a longitudinal analysis. Bone 2006;38:576–583.

30 Wang QJ, Suominen H, Nicholson PH, Zou LC, Alen M, Koistinen A, Cheng S: Influence of physical activity and maturation status on bone mass and geometry in early pubertal girls. Scand J Med Sci Sports 2004;15:100–106.

31 Janz KF, Burns TL, Levy SM, Torner JC, Willing MC, Beck TJ, Gilmore JM, Marshall TA: Everyday activity predicts bone geometry in children: the Iowa bone development study. Med Sci Sports Exerc 2004;36:1124–1131.

32 Morris FL, Naughton GA, Gibbs JL, Carlson JS, Wark JD: Prospective ten-month exercise intervention in premenarcheal girls: positive effects on bone and lean mass. J Bone Miner Res 1997;12:1453–1462.

33 McKay HA, Petit MA, Schutz RW, Prior JC, Barr SI, Khan KM: Augmented trochanteric bone mineral density after modified physical education classes: a randomized school-based exercise intervention study in prepubescent and early pubescent children. J Pediatr 2000;136:156–162.

34 Bradney M, Pearce G, Naughton G, Sullivan C, Bass S, Beck T, Carlson J, Seeman E: Moderate exercise during growth in prepubertal boys: changes in bone mass, size, volumetric density, and bone strength: a controlled prospective study. J Bone Miner Res 1998;13:1814–1821.

35 Fuchs RK, Bauer JJ, Snow CM: Jumping improves hip and lumbar spine bone mass in prepubescent children: a randomized controlled trial. J Bone Miner Res 2001;16:148–156.

36 Heinonen A, Sievanen H, Kannus P, Oja P, Pasanen M, Vuori I: High-impact exercise and bones of growing girls: a 9-month controlled trial. Osteoporos Int 2000;11:1010–1017.

37 MacKelvie KJ, McKay HA, Khan KM, Crocker PR: A school-based exercise intervention augments bone mineral accrual in early pubertal girls. J Pediatr 2001;139:501–508.

38 MacKelvie KJ, McKay HA, Petit MA, Moran O, Khan KM: Bone mineral response to a 7-month randomized controlled, school-based jumping intervention in 121 prepubertal boys: associations with ethnicity and body mass index. J Bone Miner Res 2002;17:834–844.

39 MacKelvie KJ, Khan KM, Petit MA, Janssen PA, McKay HA: A school-based exercise intervention elicits substantial bone health benefits: a 2-year randomized controlled trial in girls. Pediatrics 2003;112:e447.

40 MacKelvie KJ, Petit MA, Khan KM, Beck TJ, McKay HA: Bone mass and structure are enhanced following a 2-year randomized controlled trial of exercise in prepubertal boys. Bone 2004;34: 755–764.

41 Linden C, Ahlborg H, Gardsell P, Valdimarsson O, Stenevi-Lundgren S, Besjakov J, Karlsson MK: Exercise, bone mass and bone size in prepubertal boys: one-year data from the pediatric osteoporosis prevention study. Scand J Med Sci Sports 2006, E-pub ahead of print.

42 Valdimarsson O, Linden C, Johnell O, Gardsell P, Karlsson MK: Daily physical education in the school curriculum in prepubertal girls during 1 year is followed by an increase in bone mineral accrual and bone width – Data from the prospective controlled Malmo pediatric osteoporosis prevention study. Calcif Tissue Int 2006;78:65–71.

43 Iuliano-Burns S, Saxon L, Naughton G, Gibbons K, Bass SL: Regional specificity of exercise and calcium during skeletal growth in girls: a randomized controlled trial. J Bone Miner Res 2003;18:156–162.

44 Van Langendonck L, Claessens AL, Vlietinck R, Derom C, Beunen G: Influence of weight-bearing exercises on bone acquisition in prepubertal monozygotic female twins: a randomized controlled prospective study. Calcif Tissue Int 2003;72:666–674.

45 Witzke KA, Snow CM: Effects of plyometric jump training on bone mass in adolescent girls. Med Sci Sports Exerc 2000;32:1051–1057.

46 Seeman E: An exercise in geometry. J Bone Miner Res 2002;17:373–380.

47 McKay HA, MacLean L, Petit M, MacKelvie-O'Brien K, Janssen P, Beck T, Khan KM: 'Bounce at the Bell': a novel program of short bouts of exercise improves proximal femur bone mass in early pubertal children. Br J Sports Med 2005;39:521–526.

48 Johannsen N, Binkley T, Englert V, Neiderauer G, Specker B: Bone response to jumping is site-specific in children: a randomized trial. Bone 2003;33:533–539.

49 Specker B, Binkley T: Randomized trial of physical activity and calcium supplementation on bone mineral content in 3- to 5-year-old children. J Bone Miner Res 2003;18:885–892.

Robin M. Daly, PhD
Centre for Physical Activity and Nutrition Research
School of Exercise and Nutrition Sciences
Deakin University
221 Burwood Highway
Burwood, Melbourne, 3125 (Australia)
Tel. +61 3 9251 7013, Fax +61 3 9244 6017, E-Mail robin.daly@deakin.edu.au

Daly R, Petit M (eds): Optimizing Bone Mass and Strength. The Role of Physical Activity and
Nutrition during Growth. Med Sport Sci. Basel, Karger, 2007, vol 51, pp 50–63

....

Evidence for an Interaction between Exercise and Nutrition for Improved Bone Health during Growth

Bonny Specker[a], Matthew Vukovich[b]

[a]E.A. Martin Program in Human Nutrition, and [b]Exercise Physiology Laboratory,
South Dakota State University, Brookings, S. Dak., USA

Abstract

Exercise and nutrition are independently recognized as important modifiable lifestyle
factors essential for optimal bone health during growth. In this review, we discuss the effect
of dietary calcium, vitamin D and protein alone and in combination with exercise on bone
mass and strength in children and adolescents. Recent intervention studies in children now
provide evidence that exercise and calcium may interact with each other to enhance bone
health, but the mechanism underlying this effect is not well understood. Vitamin D is also
important for bone health through its action on calcium absorption, and both dietary protein
and total energy intake can also alter bone metabolism through their influence on growth factors such as insulin-like growth factor I. However, whether these factors act synergistically
with exercise to enhance bone accrual has not been examined. Therefore, while exercise and
nutrition are both independently important for skeletal development, there remain many
unanswered questions as to whether combinations of these factors interact to enhance skeletal health during growth. Current evidence suggests that regular weight-bearing exercise and
adequate dietary calcium intakes (around 1,000 mg per day) may be required to optimize
bone health; however, exercise would appear to be more important for optimizing bone
strength because it has a direct effect (e.g. via loading) on bone mass and structural properties, whereas nutritional factors appear to have an indirect effect (e.g. via hormonal factors)
on bone mass.

Copyright © 2007 S. Karger AG, Basel

The amount of bone gained during childhood and the rate of loss later in
life are important predictors for the risk of osteoporosis and fractures later in
life. Exercise and nutrition are independently recognized as important modifiable lifestyle factors essential for optimal bone health during growth. However,
there is increasing evidence that the beneficial skeletal effects of exercise may

only occur with adequate nutrition. Calcium and protein are recognized as two important nutrients necessary for optimal bone health during growth, and there is some evidence that these nutrients may interact with exercise in determining bone outcomes. This exercise-by-nutrition interaction is important to understand and to consider when recommending lifestyle changes in either of these factors.

Understanding the Terms 'Interaction' or 'Effect Modification'

When addressing the question of whether the beneficial effects of exercise occur only in the presence of adequate nutrition, it is important to first understand the term 'interaction'. A simple hypothetical example of an interaction was described by Hogben in 1933 and is often used to illustrate a gene-by-diet interaction [1]. The example is based on the assumption that for a chicken to have yellow shanks (e.g. legs), both a yellow shank gene and the consumption of yellow corn are required. In this example, one investigator conducts a study in a population of chickens, some of which have the yellow shank gene and some of which do not. All the chickens are fed yellow corn, and the investigator concludes that the presence of the yellow shanks is 100% attributed to genetics. Another investigator, however, studies a population of chickens that all have the yellow shank gene and half of the chickens are fed yellow corn and half are fed white corn. In this case, the investigator concludes that the presence of yellow shanks is 100% attributed to diet. This extreme example illustrates how an interaction between two factors can have significant effects on the study results and the resultant conclusions. Interactions within the context of bone exist and are discussed in greater detail below. It is important to realize that the presence of an interaction is due to relationships that are more complex, with individual factors interacting with each other. Rather than being able to separate the amount of variation within a population into individual factors whose variances sum to 100%, some of the variation attributed to one factor may be a function of how that factor interacts with other factors. For example, the variation in bone mass within a population that is attributed to diet may be a function of how dietary factors interact with specific genetic makeup, hormonal status, or even the physical activity patterns of that population. It is likely that the complexity of these interactions is one of the reasons for inconsistent findings among various studies with regard to the effect of exercise and nutrition on bone outcomes.

The presence of an interaction implies that the effects of two factors are multiplicative, rather than additive. In the example above, the outcome variable (presence/absence of yellow shanks) and the predictor variables (presence/absence of either the yellow shank gene or presence/absence of yellow corn

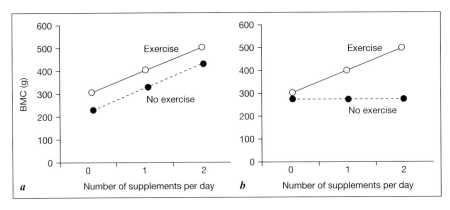

Fig. 1. a A hypothetical example of no evidence of an exercise-by-supplement use inter-action on BMC. The effect of each of these factors (exercise and supplement use) is considered additive since the level of one factor does not have any influence on the effect of the other. ***b*** An example of an interaction, or multiplicative effect, between exercise and supplement use.

consumption) were categorical or group variables. In bone studies, the out-comes are typically continuous variables, such as areal bone mineral density (aBMD) or bone mineral content (BMC). Figure 1a shows a hypothetical exam-ple of no evidence of an exercise-by-supplement use interaction on BMC. The effect of each of these factors (exercise and supplement use) is considered addi-tive since the level of one factor does not have any influence on the effect of the other. The conclusion based on figure 1a is that BMC is greater with exercise and with an increasing number of supplements taken. Figure 1b illustrates an interaction, or multiplicative effect, between exercise and supplement use. The presence of an interaction complicates the interpretation of the main effects of exercise and supplement use. In this example, it is not possible to simply con-clude that BMC is greater with exercise because the difference between the exercise and no exercise groups is not the same for all levels of supplement use. Similarly, one also cannot conclude that supplement use is beneficial to BMC since it is only true for those individuals within the exercise group. Thus, the conclusions based on the hypothetical example in figure 1b would be that exer-cise modifies the effect of supplement use on BMC (or vice versa), and that in order to benefit from one of these factors the other factor also needs to be pre-sent. If these interactions among individual factors are not considered in study designs or in the statistical analyses of data pertaining to bone outcomes, esti-mates of the amount of variance attributed to these factors are not valid [2]. Although several studies investigated interactions post hoc during the analysis stage, it is important that they are considered during the study design because the sample sizes needed to detect interactions are often significantly greater than those needed to detect main effects [3].

Combined Effect of Calcium, Vitamin D, or Protein and Exercise during Growth: Is There Evidence for an Interaction on Bone?

Bone growth in length, mass and size is dependent upon interactions between hormonal changes that are occurring during growth, as well as the loads that are placed on the skeleton, and possibly substrate availability (e.g. calcium and phosphorus). Adequate intakes of dietary calcium, vitamin D and protein are accepted as important to optimize bone health during growth, and there is some evidence that exercise may interact with some of these nutrients to enhance bone formation. Phosphorus is also important but it is present in relatively high amounts in the diets of most individuals in Western countries and low circulating phosphorus among healthy individuals is rare. The following section will review the evidence as to whether calcium, vitamin D and protein or total energy intake interact synergistically with exercise to enhance bone health during growth.

Calcium
Calcium is a primary constituent of bone and thus is recognized as a critical nutrient for optimal bone mineral accrual. Calcium requirements increase during growth, but there is some disagreement on the amount needed to optimize bone health. While it is well established that calcium is a 'threshold nutrient', there is some evidence that maximal calcium retention plateaus at intakes of around 1,300 mg per day in adolescent girls [4]. However, defining the 'optimal' amount of calcium necessary for bone health at different stages of the life span is difficult due, in part, to the complexity of how calcium may interact with other factors in determining bone mass, including other nutrients (e.g. protein and vitamin D) and physical activity.

There is a sound physiological basis for an interactive effect of calcium and exercise on bone; exercise is necessary to stimulate bone modeling and remodeling and calcium is a required substrate for bone mineralization. In 1996, Specker [5] published the results of a meta-analysis that showed a possible interaction between exercise and calcium intake on changes in spine aBMD in adults. In this analysis, which included a combination of randomized and non-randomized trials mostly involving peri- and postmenopausal women, the mean annualized rates of change in spine aBMD at different calcium intakes were examined for groups of individuals assigned to either an exercise intervention or to a control group. A total of 16 studies met the inclusion criteria for entry

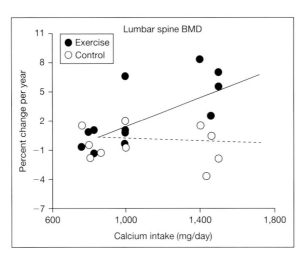

Fig. 2. Results of meta-analysis showing an exercise-by-calcium intake interaction. Taken from Specker [5].

into the analysis, with 12 studies including changes in spine aBMD. Study sample sizes ranged from 7 to 34 per group among these 12 studies. As shown in figure 2, there appears to be a benefit of exercise in preventing bone loss only at calcium intakes greater than 1,000 mg/day. Another way of interpreting these data is that the benefit of exercise on bone loss prevention only occurs when there is adequate calcium intake.

Despite the theoretical basis for an interaction between exercise and dietary calcium, there have been relatively few well-designed, randomized controlled studies conducted in children and adolescents that have tested this hypothesis. As indicated in a recent review, many studies examining whether calcium enhances the effect of exercise on bone have included both factors in multivariate analyses, but failed to report an interaction between these two factors [6]. In a study of 239 preschool children designed specifically to test for an exercise-by-calcium intake interaction [7], half the children were randomized to a gross motor activity program involving bone-loading activities (30 min per day, 5 days per week for 1 year), and the other half to a fine motor activity program that was designed to keep them sitting quietly. Within each of these intervention groups, the children were further randomized to receive either calcium supplements or placebo. The main findings from this study were that calcium intake modified the dual-energy X-ray absorptiometry (DXA) leg BMC and bone geometry in response to physical activity in young children. Bone geometry was measured by peripheral quantitative computed tomography (pQCT), which

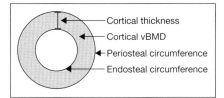

Fig. 3. Schematic of the cross-section of the shaft of a long bone, illustrating the periosteal and endosteal circumference and thickness of the cortical shell. The cortical area is shown by the gray-shaded area, in which cortical volumetric BMD (vBMD) is measured.

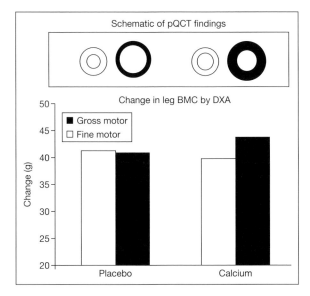

Fig. 4. The change in leg BMC shows the interaction of exercise-by-calcium intake in a randomized pediatric trial designed specifically to investigate how calcium intake modifies the bone response to exercise. The cross-sectional images above the bars illustrate the pQCT findings of the cross-section of the tibia at study completion. Taken from Specker and Binkley [7].

provides measurements of periosteal and endosteal circumferences and cortical thickness (fig. 3). These analyses revealed that gross motor activity increases periosteal circumference, or bone diameter, whereas calcium supplementation appeared to decrease the endosteal expansion that normally occurs with aging, but only among the gross motor exercise group (fig. 4) [7]. Overall, the greatest bone benefit from exercise or calcium supplementation was observed when both factors were present. Consistent with previous findings from supplementation trials, the bone benefit of calcium supplementation did not persist beyond the intervention period, while the increase in bone size with exercise was still significant 12 months after the intervention had ceased [8].

Several additional pediatric exercise-calcium trials have found results consistent with the hypothesis that greater exercise-induced changes occur in individuals with high compared to low dietary calcium intakes [9, 10]. To examine whether increases in dietary calcium intake and physical activity enhance bone mineral status in adolescent girls, Stear et al. [9] conducted a 15-month, 2×2 randomized trial among 144 females aged 16–18 years. Participants were randomly assigned (double-blind) to receive either a calcium supplement or placebo. They were further randomized within each supplement group to one of two exercise groups. The first group was asked to attend three 45-min exercise sessions a week, while the other group did not participate in an exercise program. The average attendance at the exercise classes was only 36%. A greater increase in total hip BMC among the exercise compared to the control group was observed when the analysis was limited to only those girls with more than 50% attendance (n = 76). Calcium supplementation was also associated with greater bone mineral accrual at multiple skeletal sites. The authors noted a trend toward a significant exercise-by-calcium interaction, but acknowledged that the sample size of their study was insufficient to statistically detect an interaction.

Iuliano-Burns et al. [10] conducted an 8.5-month, 2×2 randomized trial among 72 prepubertal girls aged 7–11 years whose calcium intakes were <700 mg per day. Girls were assigned to one of four groups: moderate-impact exercise with or without calcium or low-impact exercise with or without calcium. The girls assigned to the moderate-impact exercise groups participated in a progressive 20-min exercise program consisting of skipping and jumping activities performed three times per week; the low-impact exercise group followed the same format but only participated in stretching and low-impact dance activities. The supplemental calcium groups received an additional 434 mg of calcium per day supplied through food products; while the placebo groups received the same food products but without added calcium. Sixty-six girls completed the study and the mean attendance at the exercise sessions was 93% and the average compliance with the food products was 70%. A significant exercise-by-calcium interaction was detected at the femur. They also reported an exercise, but not a calcium effect, at the tibia-fibula, and a calcium, but not an exercise effect, at the arms. In a similar study conducted by the same researchers that involved 88 prepubertal boys, exercise and calcium combined (four-group analysis) resulted in a 2% greater increase in femur bone mass than either factor alone, and a 3% greater increase in bone mass at the tibia-fibula compared to the placebo group [unpubl. obs.]. The authors did not test for an interaction in this study due to the smaller sample size. Furthermore, they proposed that the lower skeletal responses in boys compared to girls may have been partly attributed to the higher baseline calcium intakes and background loading history in the boys.

Several additional pediatric trials have found results consistent with the hypothesis that greater exercise-induced changes occur in individuals with high compared to low dietary calcium intakes [11, 12]. Johannsen et al. [11] found a relationship between change in leg BMC and calcium intake among 54 children aged 3–18 years. In this study, children were randomized to either a jumping program 5 days per week for 12 weeks or to a control group. Total body, spine and hip DXA and pQCT measurements at the 4% (trabecular) and 20% (cortical) distal tibia site were performed. Overall, jumpers had a greater increase in DXA leg BMC than nonjumpers. Although calcium intake was not controlled in this study, post hoc analysis found that there was a significant correlation between the change in leg BMC and calcium intake among the jumping group, but not the control group. Although the overall sample size was small, which makes detection of a statistical interaction difficult, these findings do support the hypothesis that the bone response to exercise may be modified by calcium intake.

In a recent study by Courteix et al. [12], 113 premenarcheal girls were randomly assigned to receive either 800 mg per day of calcium phosphate or placebo that was added to milk. Although 240 subjects were initially desired, only 113 were recruited due to fears of dairy consumption surrounding mad cow disease. Each of the girls was classified into an exercise or a sedentary group based on an activity questionnaire that recorded the frequency and duration of previous sports participation. Although this was not a randomized trial of exercise, and the investigators did not test for an exercise-by-calcium interaction, the calcium-exercise group had significantly greater gains in aBMD at the total body, spine and hip sites than the other three groups after 1 year. As a result, the authors concluded that there was a beneficial combined effect of exercise and calcium supplementation on bone accretion in premenarcheal girls.

Some investigators have suggested that calcium requirements may be increased with increased physical activity. Urinary calcium excretion may be increased during intensive training, and there may be significant dermal loss of calcium through sweat [13, 14]. One study reported that urinary calcium excretion was ~70% greater following a single bout of exercise compared to urinary excretion during a control period [13], which may be related to metabolic acidosis. Calcium losses are related to exercise intensity and duration [14, 15]: running for 45 min has been shown to result in a dermal calcium loss of about 45 mg, while prolonged (>2 h) basketball practice was reported to result in dermal calcium losses of about 422 mg. The increased calcium loss due to exercise should be offset by an adequate calcium intake, and as noted above, the beneficial bone effect of exercise may only be observed if calcium intake is adequate, or at recommended intakes.

Vitamin D

Vitamin D and parathyroid hormone (PTH) are systemic hormones that are involved in the regulation of calcium and bone metabolism. PTH stimulates renal reabsorption of calcium, increases intestinal calcium absorption by increased renal formation of $1,25-(OH)_2D$, and mobilizes calcium from bone. PTH also increases the synthesis of bone enzymes that are involved in bone resorption and remodeling. Secondary hyperparathyroidism occurs with vitamin D deficiency, and it has been suggested that the serum 25-OHD concentrations below which there is an increase in serum PTH concentrations should define the lower limit of normal for serum 25-OHD [16]. In the elderly, this 25-OHD concentration is approximately 33 ng/ml [17, 18], but in children it appears to be lower [16].

Increased serum PTH concentrations or hyperparathyroidism, resulting from low vitamin D status, theoretically should increase bone resorption and decrease aBMD. However, conflicting results are observed in pediatric studies that have tried to correlate DXA-derived aBMD with serum 25-OHD concentrations [19, 20]. One possible explanation is that cortical and trabecular bone appears to be affected differently in individuals with hyperparathyroidism: decreases in cortical BMD are observed, in conjunction with increases in trabecular BMD. DXA measures of aBMD do not allow for separation of cortical and trabecular bone, which would lead to inconclusive findings.

Although the primary effects of vitamin D deficiency are on alterations in calcium and bone homeostasis, severe vitamin D deficiency at any age leads to reduced muscle strength [21]. High serum PTH concentrations observed in severe vitamin D deficiency lead to a decrease in serum phosphorus concentrations. Phosphorus is a vital component in adenosine triphosphate, creatine phosphate and other phosphorylated compounds that are necessary for normal muscle function, energy production and energy storage. In addition, there are vitamin D receptors present on muscle tissue and it has been suggested that vitamin D may have a direct effect on muscle tissue [22].

Although we are unaware of studies that have investigated an exercise-by-vitamin D interaction on bone health, it is likely that the beneficial response to exercise will not occur if secondary hyperparathyroidism exists. A recent prospective study of Finnish military recruits supports this speculation. Valimaki et al. [23] found that military recruits with stress fracture had higher serum PTH concentrations than recruits who did not have stress fracture. Although they did not find any difference between fracture groups in circulating levels of serum 25-OHD prior to fracture, they previously reported a high rate of vitamin D deficiency in this population.

Protein and Energy Intake

Over the years, it has been widely reported that a high dietary protein intake may cause excessive urinary calcium loss, negative calcium balance and increased bone loss. The primary evidence behind this originated from the proposed role of bone in acid-base balance, with theorists suggesting that the increased acid load generated from high protein intakes may require neutralization from calcium salts originating from bone [24]. While it is possible that a prolonged high protein intake may lead to increased bone resorption and ultimate bone loss, the evidence is conflicting; some studies report a beneficial effect of high protein intake [25, 26], whereas others report detrimental bone effects [27–29].

There are limited data from observational studies of malnourished children that indicate that energy and protein malnutrition are associated with reduced bone size (periosteal apposition) and cortical mass [30]. On the other hand, a recent prospective study reported a positive association between dietary protein intake over the previous 4 years and periosteal circumference, cortical area, BMC, and the polar strength strain index at the proximal radius in 229 children and adolescents [26]. The beneficial effects of protein intake appeared to be negated, at least partly, if dietary potential renal acid load was high (e.g. if the intake of alkalizing minerals was low). Therefore, despite the constant debate over the proposed action of dietary protein on bone health, there is increasing research that finds that protein has a favorable, and not detrimental, effect on the skeleton.

The positive effect that protein may have on bone is probably mediated indirectly through its action on the hormone insulin-like growth factor I (IGF-I) and its family of binding proteins, which are known to be important for both muscle and bone growth [31]. The synthesis and secretion of IGF-I is dependent upon growth hormone and the availability of adequate nutrient intake [32]; there is evidence that plasma concentrations of IGF-I and IGF-binding proteins are largely affected by both dietary energy and protein intake [33]. A recent study by Hoppe et al. [34] reported a significant positive association between protein intake, growth, and circulating IGF-I concentrations in a cross-sectional study of 90 children aged 2.5 years. Isley et al. [35] found that IGF-I concentrations decreased by approximately 60% after 5 days of fasting, while refeeding resulted in a return of serum IGF-I concentrations towards baseline. Similarly, energy balance during exercise training also has an effect on IGF-I levels, with decreased IGF-I and increased IGF-I-binding protein concentrations during 7 days of exercise training with a negative energy balance of 2,000 kcal [36]. A reduction in protein consumption with or without adequate energy intake also leads to a decrease in plasma IGF-I concentrations, resulting from either a decrease in synthesis or release of IGF-I by the liver or both. Furthermore, protein restriction may also increase receptor resistance to growth hormone at the liver or to IGF-I at target tissues.

In the study by Isley et al. [35] described above, the investigators compared the effect of low protein, isocaloric diets during refeeding on IGF-I concentrations and found that dietary protein reduction, but adequate energy, during the refeeding phase resulted in a blunted IGF-I response. At the end of the 5 days of refeeding, IGF-I concentrations in the low protein diet group were below the higher protein diet group. The difference in the IGF-I response to protein between the two groups resulted in subsequent studies focusing on the effects of protein undernutrition on IGF-I concentrations [37, 38].

In addition to the potential adverse effects of energy and protein malnutrition on serum concentrations of IGF-I and altered bone metabolism, malnutrition can also have a catabolic effect on muscle mass which can indirectly affect bone [39]. Conversely, it has been proposed that increased dietary protein may be necessary for active individuals to achieve maximal gains from an exercise program [40]. Ballard et al. [41] found in young adults that protein supplementation during a 6-month strength and endurance training program resulted in a significant increase in serum IGF-I concentrations, while the placebo group experienced a significant decrease. Although this study was not designed to detect an exercise-by-protein intake interaction, the increase in IGF-I concentrations with protein supplementation was not associated with an improvement in volumetric BMD or bone size despite an increase in markers of bone turnover. However, the short duration of this trial makes interpretation of the bone results difficult.

A recent study in ovariectomized rats reported a significant exercise-by-protein interaction on bone calcium content in those animals that were randomized to swim training or control and soy protein or control diet [42]. This interaction was observed even though the loads placed on the skeleton by swimming are thought to be less than those expected through weight-bearing activities. Although specific effects of protein intake on bone geometry during exercise have not been reported, it is hypothesized that the increase in periosteal circumference that is observed with increased loading may be attenuated in the presence of a low protein intake. However, we are unaware of any studies that have investigated a protein-by-exercise interaction on bone mass and geometry during growth. Whether a protein-by-exercise trial would likely find significant results is questionable due to the relatively high protein intakes among children in most Western countries.

Summary and Conclusion

Exercise and nutrition are recognized as important modifiable lifestyle factors essential for optimal bone health during growth. There is increasing evidence that the presence or absence of one of these factors may influence the beneficial bone effect of the other. This exercise-by-nutrition interaction is important to understand and to consider when recommending lifestyle changes. Several studies support the hypothesis that calcium intake modifies the bone response to exercise, and the use of pQCT technology has increased our understanding of the structural basis by which exercise and nutrition influence bone mass, structure and strength. Although both energy intake and protein consumption alter circulating IGF-I concentrations, the effect of dietary protein intake on IGF-I concentrations is greater than the effect of energy intake alone. However, whether protein intake modifies the bone response to exercise during growth is not known. Overall, current evidence suggests that regular weight-bearing exercise and adequate nutrient intakes are required to optimize bone health; however, except in cases of extreme nutrient deficiency, exercise appears to be more important for optimizing bone geometry and strength. Increases in bone strength through exercise can be limited, but is not controlled by, nutritional factors.

References

1   MacMahon B, Pugh TF: Epidemiology: Principles and Methods. Boston, Little, Brown and Company, 1970.
2   Rockhill B, Newman B, Weinberg C: Use and misuse of population attributable fractions. Am J Public Health 1998;88:15–19.
3   Lachenbruch PA: A note on sample size computation for testing interactions. Stat Med 1988;7: 467–469.
4   Jackman LA, Millane SS, Martin BR, Wood OB, McCabe GP, Peacock M, Weaver CM: Calcium retention in relation to calcium intake and postmenarcheal age in adolescent females. Am J Clin Nutr 1997;66:327–333.
5   Specker BL: Evidence for an interaction between calcium intake and physical activity on changes in bone mineral density. J Bone Miner Res 1996;11:1539–1544.
6   Welch JM, Weaver CM: Calcium and exercise affect the growing skeleton. Nutr Rev 2005;63: 361–373.
7   Specker B, Binkley T: Randomized trial of physical activity and calcium supplementation on bone mineral content in 3- to 5-year-old children. J Bone Miner Res 2003;18:885–892.
8   Binkley T, Specker B: Increased periosteal circumference remains present 12 months after an exercise intervention in preschool children. Bone 2004;35:1383–1388.
9   Stear SJ, Prentice A, Jones SC, Cole TJ: Effect of a calcium and exercise intervention on the bone mineral status of 16- to 18-year-old adolescent girls. Am J Clin Nutr 2003;77:985–992.
10 Iuliano-Burns S, Saxon L, Naughton G, Gibbons K, Bass S: Regional specificity of exercise and calcium during skeletal growth in girls: a randomized controlled trial. J Bone Miner Res 2003;18: 156–162.
11 Johannsen N, Binkley T, Englert V, Niederauer G, Specker B: Bone response to jumping is site-specific in children: a randomized trial. Bone 2003;33:533–539.
12 Courteix D, Jaffre C, Lespessailles E, Benhamou L: Cumulative effects of calcium supplementation and physical activity on bone accretion in premenarcheal children: a double-blind randomised placebo-controlled trial. Int J Sports Med 2005;26:332–338.
13 Ashizawa N, Fujimura R, Tokuyama K, Suzuki M: A bout of resistance exercise increases urinary calcium independently of osteoclastic activation in men. J Appl Physiol 1997;83:1159–1163.

14   Klesges RC, Ward KD, Shelton ML, Applegate WB, Cantler ED, Palmieri GM, Harmon K, Davis J: Changes in bone mineral content in male athletes: mechanisms of action and intervention effects. JAMA 1996;276:226–230.

15   Bullen BB, O'Toole ML, Johnson KC: Calcium losses resulting from an acute bout of moderate-intensive exercise. Int J Sport Nutr 1999;9:275–284.

16   Standing Committee on the Scientific Evaluation of Dietary Reference Intakes, Food and Nutrition Board, Institute of Medicine: Dietary Reference Intakes for Calcium, Phosphorus, Magnesium, Vitamin D and Fluoride. Washington, National Academy Press, 1997.

17   Krall EA, Sahyoun N, Tannenbaum S, Dallal GE, Dawson-Hughes B: Effect of vitamin D intake on seasonal variations in parathyroid hormone secretion in postmenopausal women. N Engl J Med 1989;321:1777–1783.

18   Dawson-Hughes B, Dallal GE, Krall EA, Harris M, Sokoll LJ, Falconer G: Effect of vitamin D supplementation on wintertime and overall bone loss in healthy postmenopausal women. Ann Intern Med 1991;115:505–512.

19   Kristinsson JO, Valdimarsson O, Sigurdsson G, Franzson L, Olafsson I, Steingrimsdottir L: Serum 25-hydroxyvitamin D levels and bone mineral density in 16–20 year-old girls: lack of association. J Intern Med 1998;243:381–388.

20   Vanderschueren D, Gevers G, Dequeker J, Geusens P, Nijs J, Deevos P, DeRoo M, Bouillon R: Seasonal variation in bone metabolism in young healthy subjects. Calcif Tissue Int 1991;49:84–89.

21   Pfeifer M, Begerow B, Minne HW: Vitamin D and muscle function. Osteoporos Int 2002;13:187–194.

22   Simpson RU, Thomas GA, Arnold AJ: Identification of 1,25-dihydroxyvitamin D receptors and activities in muscle. J Biol Chem 1985;72:8882–8891.

23   Valimaki VV, Alfthan H, Lehmuskallio E, Loyttyniemi E, Sahi T, Suominen H, Valimaki MJ: Risk factors for clinical stress fractures in male military recruits: a prospective cohort study. Bone 2005;37:267–273.

24   Wachman A, Bernstein DS: Diet and osteoporosis. Lancet 1968;i:958–959.

25   Promislow JH, Goodman-Gruen D, Slymen DJ, Barrett-Connor E: Protein consumption and bone mineral density in the elderly: the Rancho Bernardo Study. Am J Epidemiol 2002;155:636–644.

26   Alexy U, Remer T, Manz F, Neu CM, Schoenau E: Long-term protein intake and dietary potential renal acid load are associated with bone modeling and remodeling at the proximal radius in healthy children. Am J Clin Nutr 2005;82:1107–1114.

27   Sellmeyer DE, Stone KL, Sebastian A, Cummings SR: A high ratio of dietary animal to vegetable protein increases the rate of bone loss and the risk of fracture in postmenopausal women. Study of Osteoporotic Fractures Research Group. Am J Clin Nutr 2001;73:118–122.

28   Kerstetter JE, Mitnick ME, Gundberg CM, Caseria DM, Ellison AF, Carpenter TO, Insogna KL: Changes in bone turnover in young women consuming different levels of dietary protein. J Clin Endocrinol Metab 1999;84:1052–1055.

29   Rizzoli R, Bonjour JP: Dietary protein and bone health. J Bone Miner Res 2004;19:527–531.

30   Garn SM: The Earlier Gain and the Later Loss of Cortical Bone. Springfield, Thomas, 1970.

31   Yakar S, Rosen CJ, Beamer WG, Ackert-Bicknell CL, Wu Y, Liu JL, Ooi GT, Setser J, Frystyk J, Boisclair YR, LeRoith D: Circulating levels of IGF-I directly regulate bone growth and density. J Clin Invest 2002;110:771–781.

32   Clemmons DR, Underwood LE: Nutritional regulation of IGF-I and IGF binding proteins. Ann Rev Nutr 1991;11:393–412.

33   Takenaka A, Takahashi SI, Noguichi T: Effects of protein nutrition on insulin-like growth factor-1 (IGF-1) receptor in various tissues of rats. J Nutr Sci Vitaminol 1996;42:347–357.

34   Hoppe C, Udam TR, Lauritzen L, Molgaard C, Juul A, Michaelsen KF: Animal protein intake, serum insulin-like growth factor I, and growth in healthy 2.5-year-old Danish children. Am J Clin Nutr 2004;80:447–452.

35   Isley WL, Underwood LE, Clemmons DR: Dietary components that regulate serum somatomedin-C concentrations in humans. J Clin Invest 1983;71:175–182.

36   Nemet D, Connolly PH, Pontello-Pescatello AM, Rose-Gottron C, Larson JK, Galassetti P, Cooper DM: Negative energy balance plays a major role in IGF-I response to exercise training. J Appl Physiol 2004;96:276–282.

37   Harp JB, Goldstein S, Phillips LS: Nutrition and somatomedin XXIII. Molecular regulation of IGF-I by amino acid availability in cultured hepatocytes. Diabetes 1991;40:95–101.

38   Miura Y, Kato H, Noguchi T: Effect of dietary proteins on insulin-like growth factor I messenger ribonucleic acid content in the rat liver. Br J Nutr 1992;67:257–265.

39   Bass S, Eser P, Daly R: The effect of exercise and nutrition on the mechanostat. J Musculoskelet Neuronal Interact 2005;5:239–254.

40   Lemon PW, Dolny DG, Yarasheski KE: Moderate physical activity can increase dietary protein needs. Can J Appl Physiol 1997;22:494–503.

41   Ballard TLP, Clapper J, Specker B, Binkley T, Vukovich MD: Effect of protein supplementation during a 6-month strength and conditioning program on IGF-I and markers of bone turnover in young adults. Am J Clin Nutr 2005;81:1442–1448.

42   Figard H, Mougin F, Gaume V, Berthelot A: Combined intervention of dietary soybean proteins and swim training: effects on bone metabolism in ovariectomized rats. J Bone Miner Res 2006;24: 206–212.

Bonny Specker, PhD
E.A. Martin Program in Human Nutrition
EAM Bldg, Box 2204
South Dakota State University
Brookings, SD 57007 (USA)
Tel. +1 605 688 4645, Fax +1 605 688 4220, E-Mail Bonny.Specker@sdstate.edu

Daly R, Petit M (eds): Optimizing Bone Mass and Strength. The Role of Physical Activity and Nutrition during Growth. Med Sport Sci. Basel, Karger, 2007, vol 51, pp 64–80

....

Gene-Environment Interactions in the Skeletal Response to Nutrition and Exercise during Growth

Jean-Philippe Bonjour, Thierry Chevalley, René Rizzoli, Serge Ferrari

Service of Bone Diseases, WHO Collaborating Center for Osteoporosis Prevention, Department of Rehabilitation and Geriatrics, Geneva University Hospital, Geneva, Switzerland

Abstract

The amount of bone mineral mass acquired at the end of growth, the so-called 'peak bone mass', is considered to be a major risk factor for the occurrence of fragility fractures during adult life. Many interrelated factors can influence the accumulation of bone mass during growth, including genetics, sex, ethnicity, nutrition (e.g. calcium, vitamin D, protein), hormonal factors (e.g. sex steroids, insulin-like growth factor I), physical activity and exposure to various risk factors (e.g. alcohol, smoking, certain medications). Family and twin studies have estimated that up to 60–80% of the variance in peak bone mass is attributable to genetic factors. It can be predicted from epidemiological studies that a 10% increase in peak bone mass would reduce the risk of fragility fractures after the menopause by 50%. Intervention studies testing the effects of increasing either calcium intake or physical activity during growth provide evidence that modifying environmental factors can positively influence peak bone mass. Nevertheless, there is large interindividual variability in the response suggesting gene-environment interactions. A few studies have reported associations between some bone-related gene polymorphisms and the osteogenic response to loading or calcium supplementation. Identifying the functionally implicated genes interacting with mechanical loading and/or specific nutrients represents a formidable but hopefully not intractable challenge.

Copyright © 2007 S. Karger AG, Basel

The amount of bone mineral mass acquired at the end of growth, the so-called 'peak bone mass', is considered to be a major risk factor for the occurrence of fragility fractures during adult life. While there are many factors that can influence the accumulation of bone mass during growth, including genetics, sex, ethnicity, nutrition (e.g. calcium, vitamin D, protein), hormonal factors (e.g. sex steroids, insulin-like growth factor I), physical activity and exposure to various risk factors (e.g. alcohol, smoking, certain medications), family and twin studies have estimated that up to 60–80% of the variance in peak bone mass is attributable to genetic factors. During growth, the bone response to modification in environmental factors can markedly vary among subjects. This interindividual difference to increased physical activity or nutrient supplementation is probably, at least to a large extent, related to genetic variations modulating the susceptibility to favorably respond to environmental modifications. Scarce data suggest that polymorphisms, i.e. allelic variants of genes coding for bone-related factors, are associated with difference in the response to increased physical activity or calcium supplementation. In the general population of growing children, enhancing mechanical loading and/or increasing dietary intakes of some specific nutrients are considered as essential measures to be implemented as strategies for the early prevention of osteoporosis. However, it can be expected that these strategies are only moderately effective in large subgroups because of marked differences in the genetically influenced susceptibility to these peak bone mass environmental determinants. Therefore, it appears of great interest to identify the main genes responsible for this interindividual bone response variability. In the long term, this may eventually pave the way to personalize recommendations for improving peak bone mass.

In this chapter, we first review evidence showing the importance of bone mineral accretion (or peak bone mass acquisition) during growth, and then discuss the role of genetics and gene-environment interactions, particularly with regard to physical activity and nutrition, in bone development during childhood and adolescence.

The Importance of Peak Bone Mass

The relative contribution of peak bone mass to fracture risk has been explored by examining the variability of areal bone mineral density (aBMD) values in relation to age. If peak bone mass is relatively unimportant to aBMD and fracture risk in later life, then the range of aBMD values would become wider as a function of age during adult life. However, several observations are not consistent with such an increased range in aBMD values in relation to age. In untreated postmenopausal women, the standard deviation of bone mineral mass measured at both the proximal and distal radius was not greater in women aged 70–75 compared to 55–59 years [1]. Similar findings were reported at two other clinically relevant skeletal sites at risk of osteoporotic fractures. At both the lumbar spine and femoral neck, the range of aBMD values was not wider in women aged 70–90 years than in women aged 20–30 years [2]. This constant range of individual aBMD values was observed despite the marked reduction in spine and femoral neck aBMD values in the older women [2].

In agreement with these cross-sectional findings, a longitudinal study of women ranging in age from 20 to 94 years (median age 60 years), with follow-up periods of 16–22 years, showed that the average annual rate of bone loss was relatively constant and tracked well within individuals [3]. High correlations were observed between the baseline aBMD values and those obtained after 16 (r = 0.83) and 22 (r = 0.80) years of follow-up [3, 4]. This tracking pattern of aBMD, which is already observed during growth, appears to be maintained over six decades of adult life. This notion of 'tracking' has two important implications. First, the prediction of fracture risk based on one single measurement of femoral neck aBMD remains reliable in the long term [3]. Second, within the large range of femoral neck aBMD values little variation occurs during adult life in individual Z scores or percentiles. From these two implications, it can be inferred that bone mass acquired at the end of the growth period appears to be more important than bone loss occurring during adult life.

In a mathematical model using several experimental variables to predict the relative influences of peak bone mass, menopause and age-related bone loss on the development of osteoporosis [5], it was calculated that an increase in peak bone mass of 10% would delay the onset of osteoporosis by 13 years [6]. In comparison, a 10% increase in the age of menopause, or a 10% reduction in age-related (nonmenopausal) bone loss would only delay the onset of osteoporosis by 2 years [5]. Thus, this theoretical analysis indicates that peak bone mass might be the single most important factor for the prevention of osteoporosis later in life [5].

There is also evidence that the risk of fracture after the sixth decade may be related to bone structural and biomechanical properties acquired during the first few decades of life. Duan et al. [7, 8] calculated the fracture risk index of the vertebral bodies based on the ratio of the compressive load and strength in young and older adults (approx. 30–70 years of age). Load was determined by upper body weight, height and the muscle moment arm, and bone strength was estimated from the bone cross-sectional area and volumetric BMD [7]. From young to older adulthood, this index increased more in women (Chinese and Caucasian) than men of the same ethnicity [8]. However, the dispersion of cross-sectional area, volumetric BMD and fracture risk index values around the mean did not increase with age within a given sex in either the Chinese or the Caucasian ethnic groups [8], suggesting an important role of bone acquired prior to the age of 30. The importance of maximizing peak bone mass has also been estimated from the determination of the risk of experiencing an osteoporotic fracture in adulthood. Epidemiological studies allow one to predict that a 10% increase (about 1 standard deviation) in peak bone mass could reduce the risk of fracture by 50% in women after the menopause [6, 9–11].

Together, these findings provide evidence to strengthen the notion that maximizing bone health during growth may represent an important strategy to prevent osteoporosis and fractures during ageing. As a result, there has been considerable interest in exploring whether environmental factors can modify the genetically predetermined bone mineral mass trajectory during growth. Before discussing this possibility, the role of heredity and putative candidate genes that might be implicated in the determination of peak bone mass is presented.

Genetics and Bone Mass and Strength

Parent(s)-offspring comparison studies reveal a significant relationship in the risk of osteoporosis within families, with apparent transmission from either mothers or fathers to their children [12–16]. The familial resemblance for bone mineral mass in mothers and daughters is expressed before the onset of pubertal maturation [14]. Comparison of the degree of correlation between pairs of monozygotic versus dizygotic twins allows one to estimate more precisely the contribution of heritability to the variance of bone mineral mass [17, 18]. This computation suggests that heritability, i.e. the additive effects of genes, explains 60–80% of the variance of adult bone mineral mass. This 'genetic effect' appears to be greater in skeletal sites such as lumbar spine compared to the femoral neck [19]. It is possible that mechanical factors (e.g. physical activity, body weight, muscle force) exert a greater influence on the cortical component of the bony structure of the femur, explaining the relatively low heritability at that site. Despite the strong impact of heritability on aBMD, environmental factors still play an important role since they may account for up to 20–40% of peak bone mass variance.

Two main approaches have dominated the search for genetic factors that influence bone acquisition and thereby modify the susceptibility to osteoporosis in later life. One approach is to search by genome-wide screening for loci flanked by DNA microsatellite markers that would cosegregate with the phenotype of interest in a population of related individuals. The pedigrees investigated to date consist mainly of families with a member at either extreme of the skeletal phenotype spectrum; particularly those exhibiting either very high or very low bone mineral mass or areal density [20–22]. Genome screening for quantitative trait loci (QTLs) has also been used to detect within the 'normal' population families and/or siblings with marked differences in bone mass, size [23–25], or geometry [18, 22, 26]. The second frequently used approach is to search for an association between allelic variants or polymorphisms of genes coding for products that are implicated in bone acquisition or loss. The most studied phenotype has been aBMD or bone mineral content (BMC) because of both the ease of access and reliability of its measurement, as well as the relatively good predictability for osteoporotic fracture risk [6, 9–11]. An association between polymorphic candidate genes and fracture has also been reported [27–30]. The fracture phenotype is certainly attractive since it is the most convincing evidence of osteoporosis-induced bone fragility. However, fragility fracture is a very complex phenotype that depends not only on bone quantity and quality, but also on other endogenous factors, such as the propensity to fall, protective responses, soft tissue padding, and exogenous elements present in the living environment (e.g. electric cord on the floor, slippery surface) [31–33].

Numerous studies have reported an association between bone phenotype and polymorphic candidate genes coding for: hormones, hormonal receptors, or enzymes involved in their biochemical pathways; local regulators of bone metabolism, or structural molecules of the bone matrix [17, 18, 34–36]. Meta-analyses have been reported for the most studied polymorphisms, which include: vitamin D receptor (*VDR*) [37, 38], estrogen receptor alpha (*ESR1*) [29] and type I collagen alpha 1 chain (*Col1A1*) [28]. The polymorphisms considered in these three genes were significantly associated with aBMD, BMC and/or fracture risk [36]. However, none of these polymorphisms appear to be responsible for a substantial proportion, i.e. more than 1–3%, of peak bone mass variance. Furthermore, significant associations appear to depend upon several factors including the skeletal sites measured, age, gender, ethnicity, genetic homogeneity of the investigated population, and the interaction between genes and environmental factors (refer to the next sections of this chapter). Only a few studies have explored the contribution of these candidate genes using bone geometry or strength as an outcome. Findings from these studies are contradictory and given the small sample size, largely explained by a lack of statistical power.

One of the most interesting aspects concerning heritability of bone mass and strength is the implication of the gene coding for low-density lipoprotein receptor-related protein 5 (*LRP5*). *LRP5* is a member of the low-density lipoprotein receptor-related family coding for a transmembrane coreceptor for Wnt signaling [39]. Several lines of evidence point to *LRP5* as a candidate gene for osteoporosis. Mutation in the *LRP5* gene has been found in patients with the human osteoporosis-pseudoglioma syndrome, an autosomal recessive disorder characterized by low bone mass, spontaneous fractures and blindness [40, 41]. Interestingly, LRP5-deficient mice develop osteoporosis and sustain fractures due to reduced osteoblast proliferation and function [42]. In sharp contrast to *LRP5* mutations reducing the functional osteogenic capacity, other mutations in the same gene can lead to increased bone formation. Such a gain-of-function mutation in *LRP5* is associated with an autosomal dominant high bone mass and sclerosing bone dysplasias [43–45]. Most importantly, a QTL for aBMD in the general population was mapped at 11q12–13, the LRP5 locus

[23, 46, 47]. A population-based study of five *LRP5* polymorphisms with allele frequencies >2% found that a missense substitution in exon 9 (c.2047G → A, p.V667M) and haplotypes based on exon 9 and exon 18 (c.4037C → T, p.A1330V) alleles were significantly associated with lumbar spine bone mass and projected area in adult males, but not females. These polymorphisms accounted for up to 15% of the population variance for these traits in men [48]. Consistent with the presence of a QTL for stature at 11q12–13 [49, 50], the exon 9 variant was also significantly associated with standing height in both genders [48]. Moreover, 1-year changes in lumbar spine bone mass and size in prepubertal boys were also significantly associated with these *LRP5* variants, suggesting that *LRP5* polymorphisms could contribute to the risk of spine osteoporosis in men by influencing vertebral bone growth during childhood [48].

These observations in young healthy males led to a study investigating LRP5 polymorphisms in men with idiopathic osteoporosis [51]. This rather uncommon form of osteoporosis affects middle-aged men and is characterized by low peak bone mass and an increased incidence of vertebral fractures in the absence of any secondary causes, and by a clear heritable component [16, 52]. In keeping with the previous association study, exon 9A and exon 18T alleles were twice as common in men with idiopathic osteoporosis compared with age-matched controls (mean age: 50.4 years, range 23–70). The odds were greater than two for idiopathic male osteoporosis and fractures among carriers of the 9A-18T haplotype [51]. In a large prospective population-based study, a variant (1330-valine) of the *LRP5* gene was associated with decreased aBMD and reduced bone size (vertebral body size and femoral neck width) at both the lumbar spine and femoral neck in elderly white men [53]. In summary, these different studies suggest that some *LRP5* gene variants would increase the osteoporosis risk profile in men, possibly by influencing bone size during growth and thereby affecting an important component of peak bone strength.

Gene-Environment Interaction – Bone Response to Nutritional and Mechanical Factors during Growth

The family and personal history of fragility fractures should be taken into account by clinicians treating patients susceptible to osteoporosis. Recording these past events is a simple way to include some sort of heredity component in the overall evaluation of the risk that a given patient has of sustaining osteoporotic fractures in the future. However, to what extent a positive history of fragility fractures reflects a genetically determined susceptibility to the disease depends on other environmental risk factors. Nongenetically determined, modifiable risk factors mainly include inadequate nutrition and/or insufficient mechanical stimuli during growth. As discussed in detail in other chapters of this book, there is evidence from randomized intervention studies carried out in children and adolescents that nutritional supplementation, particularly with calcium salts, or increased physical activity can enhance the accrual of bone mineral mass. However, the bone response varies markedly from one child to another, suggesting an important role of genetic factors in the bone response to nutrition or physical activity interventions.

The findings from a number of calcium intervention trials in children and adolescents indicate that there is a marked interindividual variability in bone mineral accrual, despite recruitment of homogenous cohorts with respect to age and pubertal maturation. Furthermore, the large interindividual variability in bone accrual has been reported in both placebo and calcium-supplemented groups. In the latter group, the wide variability is found despite similar compliance among participants. This notion is illustrated in two randomized double-blind placebo-controlled trials in which the effect of calcium supplementation (850 mg/day for 1 year) was examined in prepubertal girls and boys [54, 55]. The greatest response in terms of gain in aBMD was observed at the femoral shaft. In both trials, the differences between the placebo and the calcium-supplemented group were significant ($p < 0.01$) in both the intention-to-treat and the active treatment cohorts [54, 55]. In the active treatment cohort of girls (mean age at entry: 7.9 years, range 6.6–9.4), the yearly gain in femoral shaft aBMD was 54 ± 4 and 66 ± 3 mg/cm^2 (mean $\pm$ SEM, $p < 0.01$) in the placebo and calcium-supplemented group, respectively [54]. This represented a gain of 5.3 and 6.4% in the placebo and calcium-supplemented groups, respectively. In the active treatment cohort of boys (mean age at entry: 7.4 years, range 6.5–8.5), the yearly gain in femoral shaft aBMD was 64.3 ± 4 and 76.3 ± 3 mg/cm^2 ($p < 0.01$) in the placebo and calcium-supplemented group, respectively [55]. This represented a gain of 6.3 and 8.1% in the placebo and calcium-supplemented group, respectively.

In both studies, there was a wide range of individual bone mineral mass accrual [54, 55]. In girls, the yearly gains in femoral shaft aBMD ranged from -19 to $+127$ mg/cm^2 and from $+10$ to $+122$ mg/cm^2, in the placebo (n = 53) and calcium-supplemented (n = 55) group, respectively [54]. In boys, the yearly gains ranged from -12 to $+140$ mg/cm^2 and from $+2$ to $+160$ mg/cm^2, in the placebo (n = 88) and calcium-supplemented (n = 86) group, respectively [55]. Similar ranges of aBMD gains were recorded at the other five skeletal sites measured: radial metaphysis and diaphysis, femoral neck and trochanter, and lumbar spine. However, in neither study could the marked variability in bone mineral mass accrual be explained, even to a small proportion, by interindividual differences in the spontaneous (baseline) dietary calcium consumed during the intervention year. Furthermore, in boys the large variance in aBMD gains was not significantly reduced after adjustment for both physical activity and dietary protein intake [55].

Prepuberty, compared to peri- or postpuberty, may represent an opportune time for environmental factors to modify the genetically predetermined bone growth trajectory [56]. The relatively modest effect of calcium supplementation, even at the femoral shaft, a weight-bearing cortical bone site, contrasts with the large variability in bone mass accrual observed in healthy prepubertal children. The strong influence of heritability in peak bone mass variance does not exclude the possibility that environmental factors, whether nutritional or mechanical in nature, modulate the expression of genetic susceptibility to osteoporosis. Interindividual variability in the bone response to environmental factors can have several origins in relation to an individual's genetic profile. With regard to nutrition, food ingredients may modulate the induction or expression of genes. They can also modify, by quantitative or qualitative alterations, the activity of protein gene products and their metabolites. These types of interactions would belong to the field of 'nutrigenomics' [57–60]. Nutrients may also interact with variants in the coding or promoter sequences of specific genes, thus modulating the level of expression, or the number of copies or still the function of protein products. This kind of interaction responsible for interindividual variability in the response to nutrition is supposed to belong to the field termed 'nutrigenetics' [57–60].

An interesting observation has recently been reported regarding the effect of a specific nutritional intervention to correct for a defect in skeletal development. The Coffin-Lowry syndrome is a rare X-linked disorder in which males show severe mental retardation associated with several skeletal defects including short stature, kyphosis and/or scoliosis [61]. The skeletal manifestations worsen over time. The causal genetic defect results in the inactivation of a ribosomal kinase, RSK2 [61]. One mechanism whereby RSK2 favors skeletal development and bone formation is by phosphorylating ATF4. This transcriptional factor itself regulates osteoblast differentiation during development and favors bone formation postnatally [62]. ATF4 exerts a stimulatory effect on amino acid import in eukaryotic cells [63]. Likewise, in osteoblasts this transcription factor stimulates the amino acid import [62] and regulates the synthesis of type I collagen, the main constituent of the bone matrix. ATF4 deficiency in mice results in delayed bone formation during embryonic development and low bone mass throughout postnatal life [62]. Interestingly, a high-protein diet in ATF4-deficient mice normalizes osteoblast differentiation and collagen synthesis in bone. Furthermore, both bone formation and bone mass are enhanced [64]. These observations suggest that the severe expression of genetic defect can be alleviated by simple dietary manipulation.

This model of nutrigenetics suggests that more subtle impairments in gene functions that control bone formation and metabolism could be alleviated by modification of environmental factors such as increasing the supply of specific nutrients and/or changing the type or level of physical activity. In this regard, it is also interesting to speculate on the interaction of mechanical strain and bone formation in relation to osteocyte function [65–67]. Osteocytes are terminally differentiated osteoblasts that become embedded within newly mineralized matrix during bone formation. Each osteocyte has long cell processes or canaliculi that connect other osteocytes and surface lining cells [68]. The density, distribution and extensive communication network of osteocytes make them particularly well structured to function as detectors of mechanical strain by sensing fluid movement within the bone canaliculi [65–67]. They can direct the formation of new bone by activating lining cells to differentiate into pre-osteoblasts. A key molecule implicated in this mechanotransduction process appears to be sclerostin, the product of the *SOST* gene [69–71]. Patients with sclerosteosis and high bone mass can have mutations in either the *LRP5* or *SOST* gene [43–45, 69–71]. Sclerostin can bind and antagonize *LRP5* [72], a Wnt coreceptor that is required for bone formation in response to mechanical load [73]. Mechanical loading can induce a marked reduction of sclerostin in both osteocytes and in the canaliculi network [74]. Furthermore, evidence for a key role of this molecular pathway has recently been reported by demonstrating that administration of sclerostin monoclonal antibodies to primates leads to dramatic increases in bone formation, trabecular thickness, radial, femoral and vertebral BMD as well as bone strength [75]. Therefore, genes coding for the *LRP5-Wnt* coreceptor and sclerostin are implicated in the bone anabolic response to increased mechanical strain. Polymorphisms in the *SOST* gene region that may modulate its expression have been shown to be associated with aBMD in elderly white subjects [76]. Thus, it will be of interest to explore in the future whether polymorphisms already observed in both *LRP5* [48, 51, 53] and *SOST* [76, 77] genes may be associated with variability in the bone anabolic response to mechanical loading during infancy, childhood and adolescence.

There is evidence from several studies which suggest gene-environment interactions in the skeletal responses to exercise in children and young adults. The findings from a cross-sectional study in prepubertal and early pubertal girls revealed that *Pvu*II polymorphism in the estrogen receptor-alpha *(ER-α)* gene may modulate the effect of exercise on aBMD at loaded sites [78]. Girls with the heterozygote *ER-α* genotype *(Pp)* and high physical activity had higher total body, lumbar spine and femur BMC and aBMD, in addition to greater tibial cortical thickness, than their low physical activity counterparts. Interestingly, no differences were found between the groups in bone properties at the distal radius, a non-weight-bearing site. Consistent with these findings, Remes et al. [79] reported that changes in lumbar spine aBMD following an exercise intervention were associated with the *ER-α* genotype in men who completed the exercise training. Other retrospective [80] and cross-sectional studies [81] of the *VDR* genotype have also reported variances in the osteogenic responses to loading in young adults. The *VDR* genotype was also attributed to variance in the bone metabolic response following strenuous resistance training in young adult males [82]. There is also preliminary evidence for an association between a functional polymorphism in the interleukin-6 gene and the response of femoral cortical bone area to 10 weeks of training in male army recruits [83]. Together, these studies provide some evidence that genetic polymorphisms may influence an individual's response to mechanical loading. These data are important because they open a way to study interindividual differences in the bone response to physical activity. Further, they provide new information on how the human genome can affect the relationship between mechanical loading and bone health (or vice versa).

Whether some of these genetic polymorphisms may alter bone mineral accretion in response to specific nutrients with or without physical activity is a vast research domain, which to date has received little attention. However, such an interaction has been explored in relation to calcium intake and *VDR* polymorphisms [84]. Gene-environment interactions may explain the inconsistent relationships reported between bone mineral mass and *VDR-3'*- and *-5'* genotypes [36–38, 85, 86]. Significant aBMD differences between VDR-3' *BsmI* genotypes (*BB, Bb* and *bb*) were detected in children [84, 87], but were absent in premenopausal women from the same genetic background [84]. Moreover, the latter study found that aBMD gain in prepubertal girls increased at several skeletal sites in *Bb* and *BB* girls in response to calcium supplements. In contrast, calcium supplementation had no apparent effect in bb girls, who had a trend for a greater aBMD gain than girls on their usual calcium diet with other genotypes [84, 85]. Accordingly, a model taking into account the early influence of *VDR-3'* polymorphisms, calcium intake and puberty on aBMD gain has been proposed to explain the relation between these genotypes and peak bone mass [84, 85]. The theory that *VDR-3'* alleles together with environmental calcium might exert an indirect and complex influence on peak bone mass by regulating skeletal growth remains speculative [17, 85]. Therefore, the possibility that calcium supplementation could be associated with a greater bone mass response in carriers of the *VDR* allele *B* needs to be investigated in prospective, calcium dosing trials stratifying the cohort by *VDR* genotypes [17, 84, 85]. This type of investigation will require a large investment and intricate study design. First, it would be important to start with extensive genotype screening, taking into account the low frequency of the

VDR BB allele in the general population when calculating sample size, and limiting recruitment to prepubertal girls with relatively low calcium intake (i.e. <600 mg/day). Second, it would be imperative to randomize a large number (at least ~200 per group) of those eligible participants into two placebo and two calcium-supplemented groups. The large sample size is necessary to achieve sufficient statistical power in consideration of both the large variability in bone mineral mass gain and the relatively weak effect of calcium as described above.

Summary and Conclusion

The hypothesis generated by the association between *VDR* genotype and the bone accrual response to calcium has raised the question of whether some other bone-associated polymorphisms could modulate the response to calcium or other nutrients during childhood. As already indicated, it is possible that part of the variability observed in the bone response to increased physical activity [88–92] might also be due to gene-environment interactions. While these are interesting and important questions, a study designed to answer them would be extremely complex, particularly given the evidence of a potential calcium-physical activity interaction [93–96], and the relatively small contribution of known candidate genes to peak bone mass variance. To further complicate the issue, it is thought that genetic factors (presumably factors other than those implicated in bone mass and strength) influence physical activity 'drive' and/or sedentary behavior. In adults, there is evidence for a role of genetics in habitual physical activity and sport participation [97–100]. However, a recent twin study in children compared monozygotic to dizygotic intrapair differences and showed that habitual physical activity was predominantly explained by shared environmental factors and not by genetic variability [101]. If true, this finding would slightly reduce the complexity of dissecting the various interactions between genotypes, nutrients and physical activity in peak bone mass acquisition. Nevertheless, the field of nutrigenetics or nutrigenomics regarding the susceptibility to osteoporosis remains highly complex. It appears that the genetic pathway to osteoporosis per se is likely to be a multifaceted one. It may be longer still with the putative interactions of dietary constituents and physical activity. The interplay of human genetic variation and environmental factors, from early fetal life to late adulthood, very likely modulates the risk of developing chronic diseases such as osteoporosis. Identifying the implicated genes interacting with bone-specific nutrients and the response to mechanical strain represents a formidable, but hopefully not intractable, challenge.

References

1 Davis JW, Grove JS, Ross PD, Vogel JM, Wasnich RD: Relationship between bone mass and rates of bone change at appendicular measurement sites. J Bone Miner Res 1992;7:719–725.

2 Buchs B, Rizzoli R, Slosman D, Nydegger V, Bonjour JP: Densité minérale osseuse de la colonne lombaire, du col et de la diaphyse fémoraux d'un échantillon de la population genevoise. Schweiz Med Wochenschr 1992;122:1129–1136.

3 Melton LJ 3rd, Atkinson EJ, Khosla S, Oberg AL, Riggs BL: Evaluation of a prediction model for long-term fracture risk. J Bone Miner Res 2005;20:551–556.

4 Melton LJ 3rd, Atkinson EJ, O'Connor MK, O'Fallon WM, Riggs BL: Determinants of bone loss from the femoral neck in women of different ages. J Bone Miner Res 2000;15:24–31.

5 Hernandez CJ, Beaupre GS, Carter DR: A theoretical analysis of the relative influences of peak BMD, age-related bone loss and menopause on the development of osteoporosis. Osteoporos Int 2003;14:843–847.

6 World Health Organization: Assessment of fracture risk and its application to screening for post-menopausal osteoporosis. Report of a WHO study group. WHO Tech Rep Ser 843. Geneva, World Health Organization, 1994.

7 Duan Y, Seeman E, Turner CH: The biomechanical basis of vertebral body fragility in men and women. J Bone Miner Res 2001;16:2276–2283.

8 Duan Y, Wang XF, Evans A, Seeman E: Structural and biomechanical basis of racial and sex differences in vertebral fragility in Chinese and Caucasians. Bone 2005;36:987–998.

9 Cummings SR, Black DM, Nevitt MC, Browner W, Cauley J, Ensrud K, Genant HK, Palermo L, Scott J, Vogt TM: Bone density at various sites for prediction of hip fractures. The Study of Osteoporotic Fractures Research Group. Lancet 1993;341:72–75.

10 Melton LJ 3rd, Atkinson EJ, O'Fallon WM, Wahner HW, Riggs BL: Long-term fracture prediction by bone mineral assessed at different skeletal sites. J Bone Miner Res 1993;8:1227–1233.

11 Marshall D, Johnell O, Wedel H: Meta-analysis of how well measures of bone mineral density predict occurrence of osteoporotic fractures. BMJ 1996;312:1254–1259.

12 Seeman E, Hopper JL, Bach LA, Cooper ME, Parkinson E, McKay J, Jerums G: Reduced bone mass in daughters of women with osteoporosis. N Engl J Med 1989;320:554–558.

13 Soroko SB, Barrett-Connor E, Edelstein SL, Kritz-Silverstein D: Family history of osteoporosis and bone mineral density at the axial skeleton: the Rancho Bernardo Study. J Bone Miner Res 1994;9:761–769.

14 Ferrari S, Rizzoli R, Slosman D, Bonjour JP: Familial resemblance for bone mineral mass is expressed before puberty. J Clin Endocrinol Metab 1998;83:358–361.

15 Barthe N, Basse-Cathalinat B, Meunier PJ, Ribot C, Marchandise X, Sabatier JP, Braillon P, Thevenot J, Sutter B: Measurement of bone mineral density in mother-daughter pairs for evaluating the family influence on bone mass acquisition: a GRIO survey. Osteoporos Int 1998;8:379–384.

16 Cohen-Solal ME, Baudoin C, Omouri M, Kuntz D, De Vernejoul MC: Bone mass in middle-aged osteoporotic men and their relatives: familial effect. J Bone Miner Res 1998;13:1909–1914.

17 Eisman JA: Genetics of osteoporosis. Endocr Rev 1999;20:788–804.

18 Peacock M, Turner CH, Econs MJ, Foroud T: Genetics of osteoporosis. Endocr Rev 2002;23:303–326.

19 Pocock NA, Eisman JA, Hopper JL, Yeates MG, Sambrook PN, Eberl S: Genetic determinants of bone mass in adults. A twin study. J Clin Invest 1987;80:706–710.

20 Johnson ML, Gong G, Kimberling W, Recker SM, Kimmel DB, Recker RB: Linkage of a gene causing high bone mass to human chromosome 11 (11q12–13). Am J Hum Genet 1997;60:1326–1332.

21 Devoto M, Shimoya K, Caminis J, Ott J, Tenenhouse A, Whyte MP, Sereda L, Hall S, Considine E, Williams CJ, Tromp G, Kuivaniemi H, Ala-Kokko L, Prockop DJ, Spotila LD: First-stage autosomal genome screen in extended pedigrees suggests genes predisposing to low bone mineral density on chromosomes 1p, 2p and 4q. Eur J Hum Genet 1998;6:151–157.

22 Deng HW, Shen H, Xu FH, Deng H, Conway T, Liu YJ, Liu YZ, Li JL, Huang QY, Davies KM, Recker RR: Several genomic regions potentially containing QTLs for bone size variation were identified in a whole-genome linkage scan. Am J Med Genet A 2003;119:121–131.

23 Koller DL, Rodriguez LA, Christian JC, Slemenda CW, Econs MJ, Hui SL, Morin P, Conneally PM, Joslyn G, Curran ME, Peacock M, Johnston CC, Foroud T: Linkage of a QTL contributing to normal variation in bone mineral density to chromosome 11q12–13. J Bone Miner Res 1998;13: 1903–1908.

24 Koller DL, Econs MJ, Morin PA, Christian JC, Hui SL, Parry P, Curran ME, Rodriguez LA, Conneally PM, Joslyn G, Peacock M, Johnston CC, Foroud T: Genome screen for QTLs contributing to normal variation in bone mineral density and osteoporosis. J Clin Endocrinol Metab 2000;85:3116–3120.

25 Karasik D, Myers RH, Cupples LA, Hannan MT, Gagnon DR, Herbert A, Kiel DP: Genome screen for quantitative trait loci contributing to normal variation in bone mineral density: the Framingham Study. J Bone Miner Res 2002;17:1718–1727.

26 Koller DL, Liu G, Econs MJ, Hui SL, Morin PA, Joslyn G, Rodriguez LA, Conneally PM, Christian JC, Johnston CC Jr, Foroud T, Peacock M: Genome screen for quantitative trait loci underlying normal variation in femoral structure. J Bone Miner Res 2001;16:985–991.

27 Langdahl BL, Ralston SH, Grant SF, Eriksen EF: An Sp1 binding site polymorphism in the COLIA1 gene predicts osteoporotic fractures in both men and women. J Bone Miner Res 1998;13:1384–1389.

28 Mann V, Hobson EE, Li B, Stewart TL, Grant SF, Robins SP, Aspden RM, Ralston SH: A COL1A1 Sp1 binding site polymorphism predisposes to osteoporotic fracture by affecting bone density and quality. J Clin Invest 2001;107:899–907.

29 Ioannidis JP, Stavrou I, Trikalinos TA, Zois C, Brandi ML, Gennari L, Albagha O, Ralston SH, Tsatsoulis A: Association of polymorphisms of the estrogen receptor alpha gene with bone mineral density and fracture risk in women: a meta-analysis. J Bone Miner Res 2002;17:2048–2060.

30 Garnero P, Munoz F, Borel O, Sornay-Rendu E, Delmas PD: Vitamin D receptor gene polymorphisms are associated with the risk of fractures in postmenopausal women, independently of bone mineral density. J Clin Endocrinol Metab 2005;90:4829–4835.

31 Cummings SR, Nevitt MC: Non-skeletal determinants of fractures: the potential importance of the mechanics of falls. Study of Osteoporotic Fractures Research Group. Osteoporos Int 1994;4 (suppl 1): 67–70.

32 Cummings SR: Treatable and untreatable risk factors for hip fracture. Bone 1996;18:165S–167S.

33 Schwartz A, Capezuti E, Grisso JA: Risk factors for falls as a cause of hip fracture in women; in Marcus R, Feldman R, Kelsey J (eds): Osteoporosis. San Diego, Academic Press, 2001, vol 1, pp 795–808.

34 Rizzoli R, Bonjour JP, Ferrari SL: Osteoporosis, genetics and hormones. J Mol Endocrinol 2001;26: 79–94.

35 Liu YZ, Liu YJ, Recker RR, Deng HW: Molecular studies of identification of genes for osteoporosis: the 2002 update. J Endocrinol 2003;177:147–196.

36 Ferrari SL: Osteoporosis: a complex disorder of aging with multiple genetic and environmental determinants. World Rev Nutr Diet 2005;95:35–51.

37 Thakkinstian A, D'Este C, Attia J: Haplotype analysis of VDR gene polymorphisms: a meta-analysis. Osteoporos Int 2004;15:729–734.

38 Thakkinstian A, D'Este C, Eisman J, Nguyen T, Attia J: Meta-analysis of molecular association studies: vitamin D receptor gene polymorphisms and BMD as a case study. J Bone Miner Res 2004;19:419–428.

39 Hey PJ, Twells RC, Phillips MS, Yusuke N, Brown SD, Kawaguchi Y, Cox R, Guochun X, Dugan V, Hammond H, Metzker ML, Todd JA, Hess JF: Cloning of a novel member of the low-density lipoprotein receptor family. Gene 1998;216:103–111.

40 Gong Y, Slee RB, Fukai N, Rawadi G, Roman-Roman S, Reginato AM, Wang H, Cundy T, Glorieux FH, Lev D, Zacharin M, Oexle K, Marcelino J, Suwairi W, Heeger S, Sabatakos G, Apte S, Adkins WN, Allgrove J, Arslan-Kirchner M, Batch JA, Beighton P, Black GC, Boles RG, Boon LM, Borrone C, Brunner HG, Carle GF, Dallapiccola B, De Paepe A, Floege B, Halfhide ML, Hall B, Hennekam RC, Hirose T, Jans A, Juppner H, Kim CA, Keppler-Noreuil K, Kohlschuetter A, LaCombe D, Lambert M, Lemyre E, Letteboer T, Peltonen L, Ramesar RS, Romanengo M, Somer H, Steichen-Gersdorf E, Steinmann B, Sullivan B, Superti-Furga A, Swoboda W, van den Boogaard MJ, Van Hul W, Vikkula M, Votruba M, Zabel B, Garcia T, Baron R, Olsen BR,

Warman ML: LDL receptor-related protein 5 (LRP5) affects bone accrual and eye development. Cell 2001;107:513–523.

41 Ai M, Heeger S, Bartels CF, Schelling DK: Clinical and molecular findings in osteoporosis-pseudoglioma syndrome. Am J Hum Genet 2005;77:741–753.

42 Kato M, Patel MS, Levasseur R, Lobov I, Chang BH, Glass DA 2nd, Hartmann C, Li L, Hwang TH, Brayton CF, Lang RA, Karsenty G, Chan L: Cbfa1-independent decrease in osteoblast proliferation, osteopenia, and persistent embryonic eye vascularization in mice deficient in Lrp5, a Wnt coreceptor. J Cell Biol 2002;157:303–314.

43 Boyden LM, Mao J, Belsky J, Mitzner L, Farhi A, Mitnick MA, Wu D, Insogna K, Lifton RP: High bone density due to a mutation in LDL-receptor-related protein 5. N Engl J Med 2002;346:1513–1521.

44 Little RD, Carulli JP, Del Mastro RG, Dupuis J, Osborne M, Folz C, Manning SP, Swain PM, Zhao SC, Eustace B, Lappe MM, Spitzer L, Zweier S, Braunschweiger K, Benchekroun Y, Hu X, Adair R, Chee L, FitzGerald MG, Tulig C, Caruso A, Tzellas N, Bawa A, Franklin B, McGuire S, Nogues X, Gong G, Allen KM, Anisowicz A, Morales AJ, Lomedico PT, Recker SM, Van Eerdewegh P, Recker RR, Johnson ML: A mutation in the LDL receptor-related protein 5 gene results in the autosomal dominant high-bone-mass trait. Am J Hum Genet 2002;70:11–19.

45 Van Wesenbeeck L, Cleiren E, Gram J, Beals RK, Benichou O, Scopelliti D, Key L, Renton T, Bartels C, Gong Y, Warman ML, De Vernejoul MC, Bollerslev J, Van Hul W: Six novel missense mutations in the LDL receptor-related protein 5 (LRP5) gene in different conditions with an increased bone density. Am J Hum Genet 2003;72:763–771.

46 Livshits G, Trofimov S, Malkin I, Kobyliansky E: Transmission disequilibrium test for hand bone mineral density and 11q12–13 chromosomal segment. Osteoporos Int 2002;13:461–467.

47 Carn G, Koller DL, Peacock M, Hui SL, Evans WE, Conneally PM, Johnston CC Jr, Foroud T, Econs MJ: Sibling pair linkage and association studies between peak bone mineral density and the gene locus for the osteoclast-specific subunit (OC116) of the vacuolar proton pump on chromosome 11p12–13. J Clin Endocrinol Metab 2002;87:3819–3824.

48 Ferrari SL, Deutsch S, Choudhury U, Chevalley T, Bonjour JP, Dermitzakis ET, Rizzoli R, Antonarakis SE: Polymorphisms in the low-density lipoprotein receptor-related protein 5 (LRP5) gene are associated with variation in vertebral bone mass, vertebral bone size, and stature in whites. Am J Hum Genet 2004;74:866–875.

49 Perola M, Ohman M, Hiekkalinna T, Leppavuori J, Pajukanta P, Wessman M, Koskenvuo M, Palotie A, Lange K, Kaprio J, Peltonen L: Quantitative-trait-locus analysis of body-mass index and of stature, by combined analysis of genome scans of five Finnish study groups. Am J Hum Genet 2001;69:117–123.

50 Hirschhorn JN, Lindgren CM, Daly MJ, Kirby A, Schaffner SF, Burtt NP, Altshuler D, Parker A, Rioux JD, Platko J, Gaudet D, Hudson TJ, Groop LC, Lander ES: Genomewide linkage analysis of stature in multiple populations reveals several regions with evidence of linkage to adult height. Am J Hum Genet 2001;69:106–116.

51 Ferrari SL, Deutsch S, Baudoin C, Cohen-Solal M, Ostertag A, Antonarakis SE, Rizzoli R, de Vernejoul MC: LRP5 gene polymorphisms and idiopathic osteoporosis in men. Bone 2005;37:770–775.

52 Van Pottelbergh I, Goemaere S, Zmierczak H, De Bacquer D, Kaufman JM: Deficient acquisition of bone during maturation underlies idiopathic osteoporosis in men: evidence from a three-generation family study. J Bone Miner Res 2003;18:303–311.

53 van Meurs JB, Rivadeneira F, Jhamai M, Hugens W, Hofman A, van Leeuwen JP, Pols HA, Uitterlinden AG: Common genetic variation of the low-density lipoprotein receptor-related protein 5 and 6 genes determines fracture risk in elderly white men. J Bone Miner Res 2006;21:141–150.

54 Bonjour JP, Carrie AL, Ferrari S, Clavien H, Slosman D, Theintz G, Rizzoli R: Calcium-enriched foods and bone mass growth in prepubertal girls: a randomized, double-blind, placebo-controlled trial. J Clin Invest 1997;99:1287–1294.

55 Chevalley T, Bonjour JP, Ferrari S, Hans D, Rizzoli R: Skeletal site selectivity in the effects of calcium supplementation on areal bone mineral density gain: a randomized, double-blind, placebo-controlled trial in prepubertal boys. J Clin Endocrinol Metab 2005;90:3342–3349.

56   Bonjour JP: Is peripuberty the most opportune time to increase calcium intake in healthy girls? BoneKey-Osteovision 2005;2:6–11.

57   Ordovas JM, Mooser V: Nutrigenomics and nutrigenetics. Curr Opin Lipidol 2004;15:101–108.

58   van Ommen B: Nutrigenomics: exploiting systems biology in the nutrition and health arenas. Nutrition 2004;20:4–8.

59   Mutch DM, Wahli W, Williamson G: Nutrigenomics and nutrigenetics: the emerging faces of nutrition. FASEB J 2005;19:1602–1616.

60   Mariman EC: Nutrigenomics and nutrigenetics: the 'omics' revolution in nutritional science. Biotechnol Appl Biochem 2006;44:119–128.

61   Hanauer A, Young ID: Coffin-Lowry syndrome: clinical and molecular features. J Med Genet 2002;39:705–713.

62   Yang X, Matsuda K, Bialek P, Jacquot S, Masuoka HC, Schinke T, Li L, Brancorsini S, Sassone-Corsi P, Townes TM, Hanauer A, Karsenty G: ATF4 is a substrate of RSK2 and an essential regulator of osteoblast biology; implication for Coffin-Lowry Syndrome. Cell 2004;117:387–398.

63   Harding HP, Zhang Y, Zeng H, Novoa I, Lu PD, Calfon M, Sadri N, Yun C, Popko B, Paules R, Stojdl DF, Bell JC, Hettmann T, Leiden JM, Ron D: An integrated stress response regulates amino acid metabolism and resistance to oxidative stress. Mol Cell 2003;11:619–633.

64   Sowa H, Karsenty G: ATF4 mediation of RSK2 functions in bone reveals a link between food intake and skeletal development. J Bone Miner Res 2006;21:S22.

65   Klein-Nulend J, Bacabac RG, Mullender MG: Mechanobiology of bone tissue. Pathol Biol (Paris) 2005;53:576–580.

66   Suva LJ, Gaddy D, Perrien DS, Thomas RL, Findlay DM: Regulation of bone mass by mechanical loading: microarchitecture and genetics. Curr Osteoporos Rep 2005;3:46–51.

67   Rubin J, Rubin C, Jacobs CR: Molecular pathways mediating mechanical signaling in bone. Gene 2006;367:1–16.

68   Klein-Nulend J, Nijweide PJ, Burger EH: Osteocyte and bone structure. Curr Osteoporos Rep 2003;1:5–10.

69   Balemans W, Ebeling M, Patel N, Van Hul E, Olson P, Dioszegi M, Lacza C, Wuyts W, Van Den Ende J, Willems P, Paes-Alves AF, Hill S, Bueno M, Ramos FJ, Tacconi P, Dikkers FG, Stratakis C, Lindpaintner K, Vickery B, Foernzler D, Van Hul W: Increased bone density in sclerosteosis is due to the deficiency of a novel secreted protein (SOST). Hum Mol Genet 2001;10:537–543.

70   Balemans W, Van Hul W: Identification of the disease-causing gene in sclerosteosis – discovery of a novel bone anabolic target? J Musculoskelet Neuronal Interact 2004;4:139–142.

71   Balemans W, Cleiren E, Siebers U, Horst J, Van Hul W: A generalized skeletal hyperostosis in two siblings caused by a novel mutation in the SOST gene. Bone 2005;36:943–947.

72   Li X, Zhang Y, Kang H, Liu W, Liu P, Zhang J, Harris SE, Wu D: Sclerostin binds to LRP5/6 and antagonizes canonical Wnt signaling. J Biol Chem 2005;280:19883–19887.

73   Sawakami K, Robling AG, Ai M, Pitner ND, Liu D, Warden SJ, Li J, Maye P, Rowe DW, Duncan RL, Warman ML, Turner CH: The Wnt co-receptor LRP5 is essential for skeletal mechanotransduction but not for the anabolic bone response to parathyroid hormone treatment. J Biol Chem 2006;281:23698–23711.

74   Robling AG, Bellido TM, Turner CH: Mechanical loading reduced osteocyte expression of sclerostin protein. J Bone Miner Res 2006;21:S72.

75   Ominsky M, Stouch B, Doellgast G, Gong G, Cao J, Gao Y, et al: Administration of sclerostin antibodies to female cynomolgus monkeys results in increased bone formation, bone mineral density and bone strength. J Bone Miner Res 2006;21:S44.

76   Uitterlinden AG, Arp PP, Paeper BW, Charmley P, Proll S, Rivadeneira F, Fang Y, van Meurs JB, Britschgi TB, Latham JA, Schatzman RC, Pols HA, Brunkow ME: Polymorphisms in the sclerosteosis/van Buchem disease gene (SOST) region are associated with bone-mineral density in elderly whites. Am J Hum Genet 2004;75:1032–1045.

77   Husted LB, Carstens M, Stenkir L, Langdahl BL: A polymorphism in the Van Buchem deletion region of the SOST gene is associated with increased bone mass. J Bone Miner Res 2006;21:S423.

78   Suuriniemi M, Mahonen A, Kovanen V, Alen M, Lyytikainen A, Wang Q, Kroger H, Cheng S: Association between exercise and pubertal BMD is modulated by estrogen receptor alpha genotype. J Bone Miner Res 2004;19:1758–1765.

79   Remes T, Vaisanen SB, Mahonen A, Huuskonen J, Kroger H, Jurvelin JS, Penttila IM, Rauramaa R: Aerobic exercise and bone mineral density in middle-aged Finnish men: a controlled randomized trial with reference to androgen receptor, aromatase, and estrogen receptor alpha gene polymorphisms small star, filled. Bone 2003;32:412–420.

80   Omasu F, Kitagawa J, Koyama K, Asakawa K, Yokouchi J, Ando D, Nakahara Y: The influence of VDR genotype and exercise on ultrasound parameters in young adult Japanese women. J Physiol Anthropol Appl Human Sci 2004;23:49–55.

81   Nakamura O, Ishii T, Ando Y, Amagai H, Oto M, Imafuji T, Tokuyama K: Potential role of vitamin D receptor gene polymorphism in determining bone phenotype in young male athletes. J Appl Physiol 2002;93:1973–1979.

82   Tajima O, Ashizawa N, Ishii T, Amagai H, Mashimo T, Liu LJ, Saitoh S, Tokuyama K, Suzuki M: Interaction of the effects between vitamin D receptor polymorphism and exercise training on bone metabolism. J Appl Physiol 2000;88:1271–1276.

83   Dhamrait SS, James L, Brull DJ, Myerson S, Hawe E, Pennell DJ, World M, Humphries SE, Haddad F, Montgomery HE: Cortical bone resorption during exercise is interleukin-6 genotype-dependent. Eur J Appl Physiol 2003;89:21–25.

84   Ferrari SL, Rizzoli R, Slosman DO, Bonjour JP: Do dietary calcium and age explain the controversy surrounding the relationship between bone mineral density and vitamin D receptor gene polymorphisms? J Bone Miner Res 1998;13:363–370.

85   Ferrari S, Bonjour JP, Rizzoli R: The vitamin D receptor gene and calcium metabolism. Trends Endocrinol Metab 1998;9:259–265.

86   Gong G, Stern HS, Cheng SC, Fong N, Mordeson J, Deng HW, Recker RR: The association of bone mineral density with vitamin D receptor gene polymorphisms. Osteoporos Int 1999;9:55–64.

87   Sainz J, Van Tornout JM, Loro ML, Sayre J, Roe TF, Gilsanz V: Vitamin D-receptor gene polymorphisms and bone density in prepubertal American girls of Mexican descent. N Engl J Med 1997;337:77–82.

88   Bradney M, Pearce G, Naughton G, Sullivan C, Bass S, Beck T, Carlson J, Seeman E: Moderate exercise during growth in prepubertal boys: changes in bone mass, size, volumetric density, and bone strength: a controlled prospective study. J Bone Miner Res 1998;13:1814–1821.

89   Mackelvie KJ, McKay HA, Khan KM, Crocker PR: A school-based exercise intervention augments bone mineral accrual in early pubertal girls. J Pediatr 2001;139:501–508.

90   MacKelvie KJ, Petit MA, Khan KM, Beck TJ, McKay HA: Bone mass and structure are enhanced following a 2-year randomized controlled trial of exercise in prepubertal boys. Bone 2004;34: 755–764.

91   Linden C, Ahlborg HG, Besjakov J, Gardsell P, Karlsson MK: A school curriculum-based exercise program increases bone mineral accrual and bone size in prepubertal girls: two-year data from the pediatric osteoporosis prevention (POP) study. J Bone Miner Res 2006;21:829–835.

92   Valdimarsson O, Linden C, Johnell O, Gardsell P, Karlsson MK: Daily physical education in the school curriculum in prepubertal girls during 1 year is followed by an increase in bone mineral accrual and bone width – Data from the prospective controlled Malmo pediatric osteoporosis prevention study. Calcif Tissue Int 2006;78:65–71.

93   Specker B, Binkley T: Randomized trial of physical activity and calcium supplementation on bone mineral content in 3- to 5-year-old children. J Bone Miner Res 2003;18:885–892.

94   Stear SJ, Prentice A, Jones SC, Cole TJ: Effect of a calcium and exercise intervention on the bone mineral status of 16–18-y-old adolescent girls. Am J Clin Nutr 2003;77:985–992.

95   Courteix D, Jaffre C, Lespessailles E, Benhamou L: Cumulative effects of calcium supplementation and physical activity on bone accretion in premenarchal children: a double-blind randomised placebo-controlled trial. Int J Sports Med 2005;26:332–338.

96   Welch JM, Weaver CM: Calcium and exercise affect the growing skeleton. Nutr Rev 2005;63: 361–373.

97   Perusse L, Tremblay A, Leblanc C, Bouchard C: Genetic and environmental influences on level of habitual physical activity and exercise participation. Am J Epidemiol 1989;129:1012–1022.

98   Maia JA, Thomis M, Beunen G: Genetic factors in physical activity levels: a twin study. Am J Prev Med 2002;23:87–91.

99   Christensen K, Frederiksen H, Vaupel JW, McGue M: Age trajectories of genetic variance in phys-
     ical functioning: a longitudinal study of Danish twins aged 70 years and older. Behav Genet
     2003;33:125–136.
100 Frederiksen H, Christensen K: The influence of genetic factors on physical functioning and exer-
     cise in second half of life. Scand J Med Sci Sports 2003;13:9–18.
101 Franks PW, Ravussin E, Hanson RL, Harper IT, Allison DB, Knowler WC, Tataranni PA, Salbe
     AD: Habitual physical activity in children: the role of genes and the environment. Am J Clin Nutr
     2005;82:901–908.

Prof. Jean-Philippe Bonjour
Service of Bone Diseases
University Hospital
24, rue Micheli-du-Crest
CH–1211 Geneva 14 (Switzerland)
Tel. +41 22 3829960, Fax +41 22 3829973
E-Mail Jean-Philippe.Bonjour@medecine.unige.ch

Daly R, Petit M (eds): Optimizing Bone Mass and Strength. The Role of Physical Activity and
Nutrition during Growth. Med Sport Sci. Basel, Karger, 2007, vol 51, pp 81–101

....

The Effect of Energy Balance on Endocrine Function and Bone Health in Youth

Cathy Zanker[a], *Karen Hind*[b]

[a]Carnegie Faculty of Sport and Education, Leeds Metropolitan University and
[b]Academic Unit of Medical Physics, University of Leeds, Leeds, UK

Abstract

Female athletes are susceptible to both disordered eating and menstrual cycle disturbances (MCDs). Disordered eating in combination with high energy expenditure from exercise can lead to energy deprivation. Current theories suggest that MCDs are caused by
energy deprivation rather than by exercise alone. A number of endocrine adaptations occur
with energy deprivation and MCDs, which are concomitant with imbalanced bone turnover,
reduced bone density and potentially increased fracture risk. This chapter reviews current
evidence concerning the disruption of bone metabolism that accompanies disordered eating
and MCDs in physically active girls and young women, including high-performance athletes.
Initially, an overview of the aetiology of exercise-associated MCDs and their link with disordered eating is provided. Thereafter, studies reporting changes in areal bone mineral density (aBMD) in female athletes with MCDs are considered in conjunction with change in
athletes' physical activity, nutritional status and menstrual histories. A comprehensive
overview of the disruption of bone metabolism that accompanies nutritionally related MCDs
is also provided. Emphasis is placed upon the role of energy deprivation and its endocrine
effects, which, when sustained, result in imbalanced bone turnover and low aBMD. Based on
current evidence, recommendations are made for the prevention and treatment of disturbed
bone metabolism and low BMD in female athletes with MCDs. Finally, consideration is
given to the effects of intense training and energy deprivation on endocrine function and
skeletal health in men.

Copyright © 2007 S. Karger AG, Basel

It is well documented that female athletes are susceptible to disordered eating and menstrual cycle disturbances (MCDs). These two conditions typically
develop concurrently. Disordered eating and high energy expenditure from
exercise provide the stimulus for MCDs which are accompanied by an array of
endocrine adaptations that impair health. One of the most severe and largely

irreversible health effects of these endocrine adaptations is low bone mineral density (BMD), which may reduce bone strength and increase fracture risk. The primary purpose of this chapter is to describe the disruption of bone metabolism that accompanies disordered eating and MCDs in physically active girls and young women, including high-performance athletes. The aetiology of exercise-associated MCDs and the link with disordered eating is also considered. Particular emphasis is placed upon the role of energy deprivation as a stimulus for both reproductive dysfunction and disturbed bone metabolism. In the context of this chapter, disordered eating is defined as a pattern of restrictive eating that elicits an energy deficit and concomitant adaptations of endocrine function and hormone metabolism. MCDs are classified as absent or infrequent menses that arise from the suppression of ovarian function that accompanies disordered eating.

Description of Exercise-Associated Menstrual Cycle Disturbances

MCDs in high-performance female athletes manifest as sporadic menses (oligomenorrhoea), or absent menses (amenorrhoea) [1, 2]. More subtle disturbances such as anovulatory cycles and short luteal phase cycles are also common, however these are less apparent clinically [2]. Amenorrhoea may be primary, as in delayed menarche, or secondary, with onset after menarche. Secondary amenorrhoea is usually defined as absent menses for 3 or more months [2]. In some cohorts of female athletes, including runners [3, 4] and ballet dancers [5, 6], episodes of secondary amenorrhoea may persist for many years. MCDs in female athletes aged below 40 years are usually attributable to a reversible suppression of ovarian function, which arises from a disruption of the pulsatile release of gonadotropin-releasing hormone from the hypothalamus [7, 8]. In turn, the normal pulsatile release of the pituitary gonadotropin luteinising hormone is interrupted and resumes a secretary pattern that is typical of early puberty. The magnitude of ovarian suppression may be gauged from measurements of plasma oestradiol concentration, which, in chronic amenorrhoea, approach the low levels observed before puberty or postmenopausally [3, 6]. As discussed later, exercise-associated MCDs tend to coincide with a multitude of endocrine adaptations which influence bone turnover and areal BMD (aBMD). Essential insight into the aetiology of exercise-associated MCDs has emerged from observations of the prevalence of the disorder among different cohorts of athletes, in conjunction with their physical, nutritional and training characteristics. Athletes with symptoms of ovarian suppression tend to participate in sports where a slender physique offers an aesthetic or performance-related advantage. These athletes also typically train rigorously, have a low energy intake, and a low body fat content [1, 2].

Over the past two decades, there has been accumulating evidence that energy deprivation contributes significantly to the hypothalamic disturbance of female athletes with MCDs [9–13]. There is scant evidence to support a role for exercise alone in the aetiology of such MCDs [14, 15]. Energy deprivation arises when there is failure to balance energy expenditure with an adequate energy intake. As liver glycogen stores dwindle, a fall in blood glucose concentration elicits changes in the serum concentration of a variety of hormones. These endocrine changes, which are counterregulatory to hypoglycaemia, include reductions in the serum levels of insulin, insulin-like growth factor I (IGF-I) and 3,5,3′-triiodothyronine (T_3), together with increases in serum cortisol, catecholamines and growth hormone (GH) [1, 11]. When sustained or regularly repeated, energy deprivation is accompanied by adaptations of endocrine function and hormone metabolism. Female athletes with sustained amenorrhoea have been compared to girls and women with anorexia nervosa due to similarities in physique, physiology and metabolism [1, 16]. Both groups of women present with low body mass, hypothalamic amenorrhoea, and reduced circulating levels of T_3, glucose, insulin, GH-binding protein (GHBP), IGF-I and leptin, together with elevated serum levels of cortisol and GH. This distinctive metabolic profile is associated with a disruption in the pulsatile pattern of luteinising hormone release [7, 8], along with disturbances of bone metabolism (reduced bone formation relative to bone resorption) and reduced dual-energy X-ray absorptiometry-derived aBMD. Evidence-based accounts of the metabolic link between energy deprivation and ovarian suppression are provided in two thorough review articles [1, 8].

Skeletal Parameters in Female Athletes with Menstrual Cycle Disturbances

It is well established that a considerable proportion of female athletes with MCDs display reductions in regional or total body aBMD, due to either inadequate bone gain or accelerated bone loss [4–6, 10, 17–21]. The extent of the reduction in lumbar spine aBMD in amenorrhoeic runners and dancers compared with eumenorrhoeic runners and dancers or untrained eumenorrhoeic women may be greater than 30% [5, 6, 17, 20, 21]. A reduction in aBMD may significantly increase the risk of fracture in these women. This is particularly true for underweight, amenorrhoeic athletes, some of whom fracture in response to minimal trauma [21, 22]. Indeed, the severity of low aBMD (osteopenia) or osteoporosis in some female athletes with a history of low body weight and amenorrhoea has led to a cessation of their athletic careers, a disruption in the quality of their life, and the use of pharmacological agents that are normally prescribed only for older people [21, 22]. To date, the majority of investigations of body composition, MCDs and bone health in female athletes have focused on distance runners, ballet dancers and gymnasts, probably because of a high prevalence of disordered eating and amenorrhoea in these athletic cohorts.

Some of the earliest studies of aBMD in amenorrhoeic athletes were conducted in runners in the early 1980s [10, 17, 18]. The rationale for conducting these studies was based on existing knowledge that bone loss accompanies oestrogen deficiency in postmenopausal women [23]. Amenorrhoeic runners had been shown to be oestrogen deficient, and it was hypothesised that this deficiency would explain any reduction in their aBMD [10, 17, 18]. These original studies confirmed the presence of low aBMD in amenorrhoeic compared to eumenorrhoeic runners, and thereby supported the credibility of this hypothesis. However, in the 1990s, further research provided compelling evidence to suggest that reduced aBMD as well as disturbed bone metabolism in both amenorrhoeic runners and ballet dancers were linked to an extensive, nutritionally related endocrine disruption, rather than to sex hormone deficiency alone [1, 3, 6, 11, 19, 22]. Runners and dancers with a history of amenorrhoea and low aBMD also had a history of low body weight and displayed abnormal serum levels of GH, IGF-I, T_3, leptin and cortisol. Reduced aBMD in these sportswomen was often associated with disordered eating, and in some instances, with the presence of clinical eating disorders [24].

Research published from the mid 1990s onwards revealed the limited efficacy of sex hormone replacement for the prevention or reversal of low aBMD in underweight female athletes, some of whom demonstrated a decline in aBMD when monitored prospectively [21, 22, 25–27]. However, weight gain, even in the absence of a resumption of menses, was accompanied by significant increases in aBMD, albeit insufficient to normalise bone mass [22, 25, 27]. Importantly, it was observed that low aBMD in distance runners and ballet dancers with a history of amenorrhoea was confined to specific regions of the skeleton. Most studies evaluated bone mineral content (BMC) or aBMD at the lumbar spine and hip, with the spine showing much greater skeletal deficits [20, 26, 28], which often amounted to frank osteoporosis (i.e. aBMD ≥2.5 standard deviations below the mean value for healthy adults aged 20–40 years [29]). This apparent site-specific distribution of aBMD in amenorrhoeic runners and dancers may be explained by competition between the systemic influence of hormones and energy deficiency and the local effects of mechanical loading on bone turnover [30, 31]. Under conditions of energy deprivation, systemic influences, which include changes in the circulating levels of hormones and nutrients, will tend to disrupt the balance of bone turnover in favour of bone loss [1]. Weight-bearing impact exercise may counteract this effect, but only at those skeletal sites subjected to direct loading.

Running and dancing tend to generate high vertical ground reaction (impact) forces within the lower limbs, which may help to prevent or reduce bone loss at these sites. In support of this hypothesis, studies of whole body and regional aBMD and BMC in young and adolescent female gymnasts indicate that even in the presence of disordered eating [32, 33] or MCDs [34–36], such athletes consistently display higher aBMD than their normally active counterparts [35, 37–39]. Even though puberty is frequently delayed or retarded in female gymnasts, their peak bone mass at maturity is nevertheless higher than that of untrained women of a similar age [35, 37–39]. This contrasts with young adult distance runners and ballet dancers with a history of amenorrhoea in whom the acquisition of bone mineral during adolescence at most skeletal sites, except for the lower limbs, is frequently compromised [5, 6, 19, 20].

In summary, observations from studies of aBMD in adolescent and adult female athletes with MCDs suggest that the rate and extent of bone acquisition during growth and the maintenance of regional aBMD in adulthood are governed by the balance between systemic and locally generated bone loading stimuli that accompany regular high-impact or weight-bearing physical activity. It would therefore seem that under conditions of energy deprivation, the promotion or maintenance of bone mass throughout the skeleton depends upon all anatomical regions being subjected to regular, high-impact and/or load-bearing activity. Nevertheless, it is possible that if energy deprivation is considerable and sustained for many weeks, the concomitant negative systemic influences on bone metabolism will override any counteracting effect of physical activity. Moreover, under such adverse nutritional conditions, the capacity to perform such activity and to recover adequately will most probably be impaired. This may partially explain the higher incidence of stress fractures in athletes with a poor nutritional status [6, 21, 27].

Bone Turnover in Women with Nutritionally Related Amenorrhoea

In healthy young women with normal oestrogen levels, bone formation and resorption are balanced and bone density remains essentially constant [40, 41]. Oestrogen-deficient postmenopausal women display accelerated bone turnover with excessive bone resorption leading to bone loss [40, 41]. Oestrogen treatment, which retards bone turnover, has been shown to be wholly efficacious in the normalisation of bone metabolism and the prevention of bone loss in these older women [40, 41]. The observation that exogenous oestrogen has limited

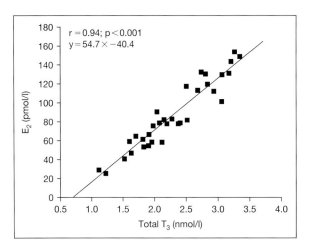

Fig. 1. Relation between serum oestradiol (E_2) concentration and serum total T_3 concentration in 33 highly trained women distance runners. Taken from Zanker and Swaine [46].

efficacy for the prevention or reversal of low aBMD in younger women with hypothalamic amenorrhoea [21, 22, 25–27, 42–45] suggests that the pattern of bone metabolism in young women with hypothalamic amenorrhoea is substantially different to that of postmenopausal women.

The first studies to characterise the pattern of bone turnover in women athletes with MCDs took place in the mid 1990s and involved highly trained distance runners [3, 46]. Runners were strategically categorised into distinct groups on the basis of menstrual patterns and the apparent magnitude of ovarian suppression, which was assessed by serum oestradiol concentration. Three groups of runners were selected and defined as eumenorrhoeic (11–13 menses per year), oligomenorrhoeic (3–4 menses per year, with a 3- to 4-month break between cycles), or chronically amenorrhoeic (failure to menstruate for >4 years). The long duration of amenorrhoea in the latter group suggested prolonged ovarian suppression, which was confirmed by reduced serum levels of oestradiol in that group. A group of untrained, eumenorrhoeic women were also recruited to act as controls. A strong positive correlation between serum oestradiol concentration and markers of energy balance in this cohort supported the idea that energy deprivation was an important contributor to their MCD [46] (fig. 1).

The most striking findings from these studies was that runners with MCDs, particularly amenorrhoeic runners, had significantly lower serum levels of bone formation markers than either eumenorrhoeic runners or controls. Furthermore, in these amenorrhoeic runners, all of whom were underweight, the extent to

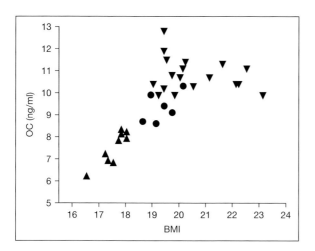

Fig. 2. Scatter plot of serum osteocalcin (OC) concentration and BMI in 33 highly trained women distance runners. These women included eumenorrhoeic runners (▼) (n = 19), oligomenorrhoeic runners (●) (n = 6) and amenorrhoeic runners (▲) (n = 9). The data suggest that in the women runners with menstrual disturbances, serum osteocalcin concentration is linked with BMI. Taken from Zanker and Swaine [86].

which serum levels of bone formation markers were reduced (relative to eumenorrhoeic runners or controls) was correlated with the degree of apparent undernutrition, which was gauged by measures of body mass index (BMI) (fig. 2), estimated energy deficit, and serum levels of T_3 and IGF-I. In contrast to previous theories, bone resorption was not elevated in amenorrhoeic or oligomenorrhoeic runners. Given the stimulatory effect of oestrogen deficiency on bone turnover, these observations of low bone turnover in oestrogen-deficient women were unexpected. These findings suggested that in underweight runners with hypothalamic amenorrhoea, suppression of bone turnover through energy deprivation overrides the stimulatory effect of oestrogen deficiency on bone turnover.

Interestingly, studies of bone turnover in young women with anorexia nervosa and low aBMD have also reported reduced bone formation [47–49]. In addition, low osteoblast numbers have also been observed in biopsies of the iliac crest of such women [50]. However, in contrast to amenorrhoeic runners, anorexic women have increased bone resorption. Recent studies of the effects of exogenous oestrogen treatment on aBMD in anorexic women have revealed little positive effect [43–45]. Importantly however, refeeding in underweight anorexic women is accompanied by an abrupt increase in serum bone formation markers, followed by a gradual reduction in the urinary excretion of bone resorption markers [48, 49, 51, 52], even prior to significant weight gain. With continued positive energy balance and weight gain, aBMD also increases, particularly if menses resume [41, 53, 54]. Collectively, these findings seem to support an essential contribution of energy balance, body weight and body composition to the balance of bone turnover in women with sustained exercise- and diet-associated amenorrhoea, and thus highlight energy deprivation as a significant stimulus for disturbed bone turnover.

Bone Turnover in Adolescents with Nutritionally Related Amenorrhoea

The aforementioned, original studies of bone metabolism in individuals with nutritionally related amenorrhoea involved young women who had probably attained skeletal maturity, rather than adolescent girls who had yet to experience the rapid phase of bone growth and mineral acquisition. In adults, a situation wherein bone formation is reduced and bone turnover is uncoupled in favour of increased resorption will ultimately lead to bone loss. In children and adolescents however, this imbalance of bone turnover will culminate in reduced bone growth and mineral acquisition. Indeed, if bone formation is suppressed and/or bone resorption is enhanced during a rapid phase of skeletal growth and bone mineral accrual, the capacity to achieve normal adult bone size and mass may be permanently impaired. Thus, the presence of nutritionally related primary or secondary amenorrhoea prior to the attainment of skeletal maturity should be treated seriously by health care professionals.

To date, there have been no detailed studies of bone metabolism in adolescent female athletes with primary or secondary amenorrhoea. However, an insight into the disturbance of bone turnover in active, energy-deprived adolescents with amenorrhoea has recently emerged from studies of patients with anorexia nervosa. Osteopenia has been observed in over 50% of adolescent girls with diagnosed anorexia nervosa [41, 53, 55, 56]. In a case-controlled cross-sectional study, Soyka et al. [57] assessed bone metabolism in patients with anorexia who were matched to healthy girls of a similar chronological age (15.5–16.0 years) and maturity (bone age). The main finding from this study was that serum concentrations of the bone formation markers osteocalcin and bone-specific alkaline phosphatase (BAP) were significantly lower in anorexic adolescents than healthy controls. There was also a trend towards a lower urinary excretion of the bone resorption markers deoxypyridinoline and N-telopeptide (NTX) when normalised to creatinine excretion in the anorexic group. Subsequent cross-sectional comparative studies of bone metabolism in anorexic adolescents and their healthy counterparts have also demonstrated lower bone turnover in the anorexic group relative to controls [51, 52, 58].

There have been few longitudinal studies of bone turnover in conjunction with changes in aBMD in adolescent girls with anorexia nervosa. However, two studies [52, 59], which employed refeeding as part of a programme of rehabilitation, demonstrated significant increases in all markers of bone formation (which were reduced before the intervention) over a 6- to 12-month period of treatment. Soyka et al. [59] followed 19 anorexic adolescents and 19 healthy controls matched for bone age and chronological age (mean ± SE, age 15.4 ± 0.4 years) over a period of 12 months of out-patient therapy. At baseline, the mean (± SE) BMI was 16.5 ± 0.4 and the mean duration of illness was 19 ± 5 months. Lumbar spine aBMD was more than 1 SD below the mean values measured in controls in 42% of anorexic patients, and more than 2 SD below the mean in 16% of patients. The most significant determinant of aBMD at this measurement site was the duration of illness (r = −0.58; p = 0.008). During follow-up, 11 of the anorexic patients recovered their body weight and 8 of these 11 girls also resumed regular menses.

The body-weight-recovered patients showed marked increases in bone turnover, with an average 75–80% increase in serum osteocalcin and BAP, and a 90% increase in urinary NTX. After 12 months of treatment, bone marker measurements were similar in the anorexic and control groups. In contrast, the 8 non-recovered anorexic patients displayed a 15–20% reduction in serum osteocalcin and BAP, in conjunction with a near 20% decrease in normalised urinary NTX excretion. These changes suggested that sustained anorexia nervosa is associated with a progressive reduction in bone turnover. Control subjects displayed the anticipated 10–20% decline in bone turnover that is normal for healthy girls after menarche [57, 59].

Interestingly, despite an increase in bone turnover in recovered anorexic patients, which normalised their serum levels of bone formation and resorption markers, the group as a whole showed no significant change in either BMC or aBMD at any measured site. The percentage change in lumbar spine aBMD of weight-recovered patients ranged from −3.1 to +9.2%; however, in none of these patients did the lumbar spine aBMD z-score increase from below −1 SD to above −1 SD. This contrasted with the changes in lumbar spine aBMD in all controls, which ranged from +0.1 to 18.8%. Within the anorexic group as a whole (both recovered and non-recovered), gains in aBMD at the lumbar spine were predicted by an increase in lean body mass (r = 0.62; p = 0.008) and by an increase in the normalised urinary excretion of NTX (r = 0.53; p = 0.05). The greatest increases in lumbar spine aBMD with weight gain were observed in anorexic girls who initially had delayed maturation (bone age) and primary amenorrhoea. This finding concurs with data describing increases in aBMD with weight gain in ballet dancers with either primary or secondary amenorrhoea [22].

Heer et al. [51, 52] also observed significant increases in bone turnover markers in response to positive energy balance and weight gain in anorexic adolescent girls throughout 15 weeks of in-patient treatment. These girls were slightly younger than those in the study of Soyka et al. [59] with a mean ($\pm$ SE) age of 14.1 ± 0.3 years at baseline, a mean BMI of 14.2 ± 0.4, and a mean duration of illness of 11.4 ± 0.4 months. When compared to a group of healthy controls, serum levels of the bone formation markers BAP and carboxy-terminal propeptide of type 1 collagen (P1CP) were both reduced by around 50% in anorexic patients, which resulted in significant differences between the two groups (BAP: $p = 0.001$; P1CP: $p = 0.007$). These bone formation markers increased significantly over 15 weeks of refeeding to reach levels that were similar to those of controls. In contrast, the serum bone resorption marker C-telopeptide (CTX) did not differ between anorexic patients and controls, either at baseline or during refeeding, although it decreased significantly in the anorexic group with refeeding. Importantly, within this particular study, changes in bone turnover in both groups were monitored for another 35 weeks after discharge of the anorexic group from hospital. During this time, 13 of the 19 anorexic patients lost weight; however, the majority managed to retain most of the weight they had gained during in-patient treatment. Through the out-patient phase of treatment, serum levels of BAP and P1CP decreased, but not significantly, and serum CTX concentration showed little change and did not differ from controls. No measures of aBMD were reported in this study. Figure 3 illustrates fluctuations of bone markers over the 50-week study in patients and controls.

Together, these longitudinal studies of skeletal parameters in anorexic adolescents demonstrate the marked effect of gross changes in energy balance, body mass and body composition on markers of bone turnover in adolescent girls and the capacity to accrue bone mass. The findings highlight the potential for sustained energy deprivation during childhood and adolescence to diminish bone growth, skeletal maturation and skeletal integrity. Certainly, studies in young women with a history of anorexia during adolescence have invariably demonstrated the presence of osteopenia or osteoporosis in these women [1, 42, 60]. Clearly, low BMC, aBMD and bone size in adolescents with anorexia nervosa are concomitant with reduced bone turnover and a dominant reduction of bone formation. Moreover, gains in these skeletal parameters with nutritional rehabilitation do not appear to be immediate.

The severity of the reductions of aBMD in anorexic adolescents has been shown to depend upon the duration of the illness and the age of its onset [55–57, 61]. It would appear that the earlier the onset of chronic anorexia nervosa in relation to the extent of skeletal maturation, the poorer the prognosis for future bone strength. Moreover, progression of the illness beyond the second decade is often accompanied by further bone loss [42, 54]. Conversely, recovery

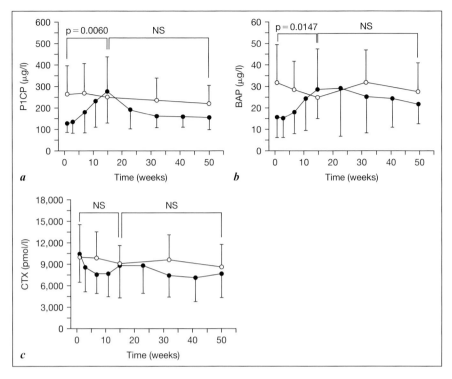

Fig. 3. Mean (± SD) serum concentrations of the bone formation markers P1CP (*a*) and BAP (*b*) and the bone resorption marker CTX (*c*) in 19 adolescent patients with anorexia nervosa (●) and in 19 age-matched healthy control subjects (○) during 1 year of nutritional therapy. Statistical analysis involved repeated-measures analysis of covariance with age and menstrual status as covariates. The p values represent the interactions between the patients and the control subjects during the respective periods. Taken from Heer et al. [52].

of body weight and menstrual function in anorexic adolescents [59, 62] and young adults [42, 53] may be accompanied by significant bone gain, and in some instances by the reversal of osteopenia.

The extent to which data describing bone metabolism in anorexic adolescents apply to adolescent athletes with amenorrhoea can only be speculated and we must await the conduct of longitudinal studies which track changes in bone turnover, BMC and aBMD in such athletes. The behavioural focus that underlies energy deprivation may be dissimilar in anorexia and adolescent athletes, but given the comparable aetiology of the MCD in these two groups and the accompanying metabolic aberrations, a common mechanism may be assumed. As with the anorexic adolescent, there is evidence for an improvement in bone health of the underweight, amenorrhoeic teenage athlete with sustained positive energy balance [6].

Proposed Mechanisms of Disturbed Bone Turnover under Conditions of Energy Deprivation

Following the observation in the mid 1990s of reduced bone turnover in women with sustained, nutritionally related amenorrhoea, research has since focused on identifying the underlying mechanisms. The key findings from this work indicate that adaptations in endocrine function in relation to energy deprivation are the likely driving force for low bone turnover and in particular, reduced bone formation in both amenorrhoeic athletes and anorexic women. Of the array of endocrine changes that accompany energy deprivation, reductions in the synthesis and serum levels of IGF-I and leptin, together with impaired IGF-I action have emerged as primary stimuli for disturbed bone turnover [3, 47–49, 51, 52, 57, 59, 63].

Reduced Synthesis and Action of Insulin-Like Growth Factor I in Energy Deprivation

IGF-I is a peptide hormone that is synthesised by many peripheral tissues in response to the action of GH and is released to serum in line with its rate of synthesis. There is substantial evidence that IGF-I mediates the anabolic effects of GH in most tissues, acting through endocrine, paracrine and autocrine actions [64]. In bone, IGF-I acts on osteoblasts and pre-osteoblasts, which stimulates osteoblast production and the synthesis of type 1 collagen [64, 65]. Thus, IGF-I is an important stimulator of bone formation, and a reduction of its synthesis in bone, or a decline in serum IGF-I concentration are concomitant with reduced bone formation [1, 65]. Acute and chronic energy deprivation, as well as specific protein deprivation are accompanied by a reduction in the serum concentration of IGF-I [64, 65]. Energy deprivation inevitably leads to negative nitrogen balance, and the magnitude of the reduction in serum IGF-I concentration during energy deprivation is closely related to the extent of negative nitrogen balance [64, 65].

The primary mechanism through which energy deprivation reduces serum IGF-I concentration is thought to involve a reduction in the density of GH receptors on the cell surfaces of peripheral tissues, including bone [64, 65]. This results in GH resistance, which is characterised by a decline in the synthesis of IGF-I and a lower release of IGF-I to serum. Keto-acidosis during energy deficit compounds the effects of GH resistance and induces a negative calcium balance as bone mineral degrades to release calcium ions for the buffering of excess protons [66]. In addition, there is an increased rate of IGF-I clearance from serum during energy deprivation [64, 65]. Furthermore, the endocrine action of circulating IGF-I is reduced in association with alterations in the serum levels of IGF-binding proteins (IGFBPs); in particular, an increase in the serum concentration of IGFBP-I [64, 67]. The IGFBPs transport IGF-I in serum and regulate the biological activity of IGF-I. Whereas IGFBP-III appears to augment IGF-I activity, IGFBP-II and IGFBP-I inhibit it [64]. The extent of GH resistance during energy deprivation is related to the magnitude of the reduction in the serum concentration of GHBP, which reflects the extracellular domain of hepatic GH receptors [64, 68]. Thus, a lowered serum concentration of GHBP probably marks a reduced density of cell surface GH receptors within the liver, the organ within which the majority of serum IGF-I is derived.

In women with anorexia nervosa, there appears to be a broad disruption of the peripheral action of GH. Reduced serum concentration of IGF-I is typical in this population, and is usually accompanied by reduced serum levels of GHBP and IGFBP-III alongside elevated serum levels of IGFBP-I and IGFBP-II [68, 69]. Comparable alterations in the circulating balance of the IGFBPs have been observed in amenorrhoeic runners [12, 70]. Indeed, the first comparative studies of bone turnover in runners with amenorrhoea or eumenorrhoea and untrained controls demonstrated reduced bone formation, together with reduced serum levels of IGF-I (and reduced T_3, a marker of energy deprivation) in amenorrhoeic runners [1, 3]. Furthermore, in these amenorrhoeic runners, linear relationships were observed between the bone formation markers and IGF-I.

Insulin-Like Growth Factor I and Bone Turnover in Nutritionally Related Amenorrhoea

A number of studies have shown that girls and women with anorexia nervosa have both reduced bone formation markers and serum IGF-I levels [47–49, 57, 59, 63]. In most of these studies, osteocalcin was measured as the key bone formation marker and was, on average, 30–40% lower in anorexic patients than healthy controls. In the same women, serum IGF-I was 40–60% lower. These differences in osteocalcin and IGF-I between anorexic women and controls compare with the 30–35% reductions reported in amenorrhoeic runners relative to eumenorrhoeic runners or untrained eumenorrhoeic controls [3]. Significant positive relationships between bone formation markers and IGF-I have also been documented in both women and adolescent girls with anorexia nervosa [65, 56]. Furthermore, refeeding of anorexic patients has been shown to be accompanied by abrupt increases in both bone formation markers and IGF-I [48, 49, 51, 52].

Indeed, Hotta et al. [49] reported a 7-fold increase in serum IGF-I in 8 severely malnourished anorexic women (BMI < 14.5) after only 3 days of intensive refeeding. After the completion of 7 days of refeeding, serum osteocalcin had increased by a mean value of 34% in these patients, while after 21 days, levels had attained values equivalent to that measured within healthy controls. In a study of adolescent anorexic girls who recovered their body weight, Soyka et al. [59] also showed that over 12 months of out-patient treatment serum levels of both IGF-I and bone turnover markers had normalised. In addition, changes in IGF-I levels over 12 months of treatment were strongly correlated with changes in osteocalcin ($r = 0.77$; $p < 0.001$) and deoxypyridinoline ($r = 0.66$; $p < 0.01$). Heer et al. [51, 52] reported a 2-fold increase in the serum bone formation marker P1CP and a 3-fold increase in IGF-I, concomitant with an increase in BMI from 14.2 ± 1.4 to 17.1 ± 0.7 over 11 weeks in 19 anorexic adolescent girls. Together, these findings suggest a profound effect of a reversal of energy deprivation on both the synthesis of IGF-I and the balance of bone turnover.

In accordance with the link between energy balance, IGF-I and bone formation, the protection of bone mass may be assisted under conditions of energy deprivation if a normal level of IGF-I activity is maintained. This hypothesis is supported by the studies of Grinspoon et al. [44, 47], which demonstrated that reduced serum bone formation markers in anorexic women may be reversed by the subcutaneous administration of recombinant human IGF-I (rhIGF-I) without a reversal of energy deprivation. Moreover, in one of these studies [44], a significant (1.8%) increase in lumbar spine aBMD was observed in a group of anorexic women treated with rhIGF-I together with an oral contraceptive over a 9-month period. In this same study, rhIGF-I treatment alone did not significantly increase aBMD. Anorexic women treated with oral contraceptive alone or a placebo lost bone mineral. These findings indicate that in anorexic women, a combined treatment strategy that enhances bone formation and reduces bone resorption may assist in the stabilisation of bone turnover. Interestingly, short-term intervention studies involving deliberate energy deprivation have also demonstrated a concomitant suppression of bone formation and a reduction in serum IGF-I levels of a comparable magnitude to that typically reported in healthy, physically active individuals [71, 72]. Collectively, these studies provide convincing evidence to support an important trophic effect of IGF-I within bone and serve to illustrate the deleterious effects of a deficiency of this growth factor on bone metabolism.

Serum Leptin Concentration and Bone Metabolism

Over recent years, reduced plasma leptin concentration has been linked with disturbed bone turnover and bone loss under conditions of energy deprivation

[52, 78]. Leptin has been designated to have a number of physiological roles, which include the neuro-endocrine control of gonadal function, the regulation of appetite, the initiation of a number of endocrine responses to energy deprivation and the direct control of bone cell differentiation [73–76]. Indeed, it is possible that a function of leptin is to regulate bone mass concurrently with changes in body mass. Plasma leptin levels are significantly reduced in lean women with nutritionally related amenorrhoea, and the normal diurnal variation is absent [73, 74].

Leptin has been shown to exert a direct osteotrophic effect in vitro. First, it acts upon the human marrow stromal cell line to enhance osteoblast generation via an inhibition of adipocyte differentiation [75]. Second, it inhibits osteoclast generation [76]. However, it has also been suggested that leptin regulates bone turnover through a central pathway subsequent to binding to its specific receptors located on hypothalamic nuclei, the effect of which may be to reduce bone formation [77]. Even so, there is clear evidence that the increase in plasma leptin concentration that accompanies the reversal of energy deprivation in anorexia nervosa patients coincides with a positive balance of bone turnover. For example, Heer et al. [52] demonstrated a dose-dependent increase in bone formation markers, leptin and IGF-I with refeeding and weight gain in anorexic adolescents. Over 15 weeks of in-patient treatment, plasma leptin levels increased over 3-fold to reach levels that were close to those of healthy controls [52]. Furthermore, subsequent weight loss led to proportionate decreases in these same metabolic variables. Of particular importance, treatment of young women with nutritionally related amenorrhoea with recombinant human leptin over a 3-month period, which led to an approximate 11-fold increase in plasma leptin concentration, not only restored ovulatory menstrual cycles without weight gain, but increased markers of bone formation (osteocalcin and BAP) compared to pretreatment values [78].

Effect of Intense Training on Endocrine Function and Bone Health in Young Male Athletes

There have been few studies that have investigated the effects of intense endurance training on bone metabolism or aBMD in boys or men. A small number of studies have reported lower aBMD in adult male distance runners [28, 79–81] and cyclists [82, 83] relative to sedentary controls. The earliest of these studies [79, 81] reported lower serum testosterone levels in runners compared with untrained men. However, testosterone levels were not depressed beyond the lower limit of the normal range for healthy men. Furthermore, there was no relationship between serum testosterone levels and aBMD of the lumbar spine. More recently, studies have linked low spine aBMD with energy deprivation in male distance runners [28]. Interestingly, this same study showed a similar prevalence and magnitude of low lumbar spine aBMD in equally trained male and female distance runners. None of these runners displayed low aBMD at the hip, probably because of a protective mechanical loading effect of running within the lower limbs. Acute, short-term (3 days) energy deprivation in male distance runners has been shown to result in significant reductions of a comparable magnitude in the serum levels of both the N-terminal propeptide of type 1 collagen, a bone formation marker, and IGF-I [71]. Currently, there is little evidence to suggest that intensive training delays puberty or skeletal growth in adequately nourished boys [84, 85]. This is despite observations that in peripubertal male gymnasts, lower IGF-I to cortisol ratios have been observed after periods of strenuous training [84].

Recommendations for the Prevention and Treatment of Low Bone Density in Female Athletes

There is strong evidence that MCDs in athletes and related changes in bone turnover are largely due to energy deprivation and subsequent effects on endocrine function and body composition. On the basis of this evidence, the maintenance (or restoration) of energy balance in lean, physically active individuals (males or females) is essential for the prevention of deficits in bone acquisition during growth, or untimely bone loss in young adulthood. Dietary intakes of carbohydrate and protein should also be sufficient to replace glycogen and prevent the loss of muscle tissue. The most effective treatment for disturbed bone turnover and reduced aBMD in undernourished, physically active individuals is to restore a positive energy balance that leads to weight gain.

Superficially, the prevention of low aBMD in athletes is straightforward, but in reality, the avoidance of energy deprivation presents more of a challenge. Most athletes are sensitive to a possible influence of 'excess' body fat on performance and may therefore struggle to achieve a balance between maintaining an optimal degree of leanness whilst simultaneously preserving their health. Indeed, it could be speculated that for some athletes, outstanding performance in their sport and good health are incompatible. Women with a low BMI and amenorrhoea may request advice on the magnitude of weight gain necessary to reverse the endocrine disturbances that underpin their low aBMD. It is probably unrealistic to establish a target body mass for any individual that equates to balanced bone turnover because of the many factors that influence bone metabolism, such as age, genetics, diet, type of regular exercise and body composition. Nevertheless, the presence of regular menses tends to signal an endocrine balance. This normally coincides with a BMI >19.5 or body fat $>21\%$ in women [1]; however, these figures may differ for adolescent girls.

At present, there is scant evidence that drug treatment is efficacious for the prevention or treatment of low aBMD associated with energy deprivation in adolescent girls or young adult women. When energy is deprived, the use of combined oestrogen and progestin treatment has been shown to confer little protection to the skeleton [22, 25, 42, 43–45]. Although combined rhIGF-I and oral contraceptive treatment [44], as well as treatment with recombinant human leptin [78] have been shown to stimulate bone formation, further research is required before these treatments may be considered for routine use in this age group. There is some evidence to support the efficacy of high-impact and weight-bearing activity for the promotion of bone mineral acquisition and the preservation of bone mass within loaded regions of the skeleton of energy-deprived individuals [34–39]; however, it should be acknowledged that site-specific osteogenic stimuli compete with systemic perturbations to the balance of bone turnover. Moreover, engagement in high-impact and weight-bearing activity may increase the risk of fracture in individuals with established osteoporosis. We recommend that coaches of young athletes, their parents and the athletes themselves be provided with clear information regarding the potential consequences of energy deprivation on bone health.

References

1   Zanker CL, Cooke CB: Energy balance, endocrine function and bone health. Med Sci Sports Exerc 2004;36:1372–1381.
2   Redman L, Loucks AB: Menstrual disorders in athletes. Sports Med 2005;35:747–755.
3   Zanker CL, Swaine IL: Bone turnover in amenorrhoeic and eumenorrhoeic women distance runners. Scand J Med Sci Sports 1998;8:20–26.
4   Burrows M, Nevill AM, Bird S, Simpson D: Physiological factors associated with low bone mineral density in female endurance runners. Br J Sports Med 2003;37:67–71.
5   Valentino R, Savastano S, Tommaselli AP, D'Amore G, Dorato A, Lombardi G: The influence of intense ballet training on trabecular bone mass, hormone status and gonadotropin structure in young women. J Clin Endocrinol Metab 2001;86:4674–4678.
6   Warren MP, Brooks-Gunn J, Fox RP, Holderness CC, Hyle EP, Hamilton WG: Osteopenia in exercise-associated amenorrhea using ballet dancers as a model: a longitudinal study. J Clin Endocrinol Metab 2002;87:3162–3168.
7   Veldhuis JD, Evans WS, Demers LM: Altered neuroendocrine regulation of gonadotropin secretion in women distance runners. J Clin Endocrinol Metab 1985;61:557–563.
8   Zanker CL: The regulation of reproductive function in athletic women: an investigation of the roles of energy availability and body composition. Br J Sports Med 2006;40:489–490.
9   Warren MP: The effects of exercise on pubertal progression and reproductive function in girls. J Clin Endocrinol Metab 1980;51:1150–1157.
10 Marcus R, Cann C, Madvig P, Minkoff J, Goddard M, Bayer M: Menstrual function and bone mass in elite distance runners. Ann Intern Med 1985;102:158–163.
11 Myerson M, Gutin B, Warren MP, May MT, Contento I, Lee M: Resting metabolic rate and energy balance in amenorrheic and eumenorrheic runners. Med Sci Sport Exerc 1991;23:15–22.

12 Laughlin GA, Yen SSC: Nutritional and endocrine-metabolic aberrations in amenorrheic athletes. J Clin Endocrinol Metab 1996;81:4301–4309.

13 Loucks AB, Verdun M, Heath EM: Low energy availability, not the stress of exercise alters LH pulsatility in exercising women. J Appl Physiol 1998;84:37–46.

14 Rogel AD, Weltman A, Weltman JY: Durability of the reproductive axis in eumenorrheic women during 1 year of endurance training. J Appl Physiol 1992;72:1571–1580.

15 Williams NI, Helmreich DL, Parfitt DB, Caston-Balderrama A, Cameron JL: Evidence for a causal role of low energy availability in the induction of menstrual cycle disturbances during strenuous exercise training. J Clin Endocrinol Metab 2001;86:5184–5193.

16 De Souza MJ, Metzger DA: Reproductive dysfunction in amenorrheic athletes and anorexic patients: a review. Med Sci Sports Exerc 1991;23:995–1007.

17 Drinkwater BL, Nilson K, Chestnut CH 3rd, Bremner WJ, Shainholtz S, Southworth MB: Bone mineral content of amenorrheic and eumenorrheic athletes. N Engl J Med 1984;311:277–281.

18 Cann CE, Martin MC, Genant HK, Jaffe RB: Decreased spinal mineral content of amenorrheic women. JAMA 1984;251:626–629.

19 Myburgh KH, Bachrach LK, Lewis B, Kent K, Marcus R: Low BMD at axial and appendicular sites in amenorrheic athletes. Med Sci Sports Exerc 1993;25:1197–1202.

20 Micklesfield LK, Lambert EV, Fataar AB, Noakes TD, Myburgh KH: Bone mineral density in mature, pre-menopausal ultramarathon runners. Med Sci Sports Exerc 1995;27:688–696.

21 Zanker CL, Cooke CB, Oldroyd B, Truscott JG, Jacobs HS: Annual changes of bone density over 12 years in an amenorrheic athlete. Med Sci Sports Exerc 2004;36:137–142.

22 Warren MP, Brooks-Gunn J, Fax RP, Holderness CC, Hyle EP, Hamilton WG, Hamilton L: Persistent osteopenia in ballet dancers with amenorrhea and delayed menarche despite hormone therapy: a longitudinal study. Fertil Steril 2003;80:398–404.

23 Worley RJ: Age, estrogen, and bone density. Clin Obstet Gynecol 1981;24:203–218.

24 Otis CL, Drinkwater B, Johnson M, Loucks AB, Wilmore J: American College of Sports Medicine position stand: the Female Athlete Triad. Med Sci Sports Exerc 1997;29:i–ix.

25 Hergenroeder AC: Bone mineralisation, hypothalamic amenorrhea and sex steroid therapy in female adolescents and young adults. J Pediatr 1995;126:683–689.

26 Gremion GR, Rizzoli D, Slosman G, Theintz G, Bonjour JP: Oligo-amenorrheic long-distance runners may lose more bone in spine than femur. Med Sci Sports Exerc 2001;33:15–21.

27 Drinkwater BL, Nilson K, Ott S, Chestnut CH: Bone mineral density after resumption of menses in amenorrheic athletes. JAMA 1986;256:380–382.

28 Hind K, Evans AJ, Truscott JG: Low lumbar spine bone mineral density in both male and female endurance runners. Bone 2006;39:880–885.

29 Kanis JA, Melton U, Christiansen C, Johnston CC, Khaltaev N: The diagnosis of osteoporosis. J Bone Miner Res 1994;9:1137–1141.

30 Frost HM: Skeletal structural adaptations to mechanical usage (SATMU). Re-defining Wolff's law: the bone modeling problem. Anat Rec 1990;226:403–422.

31 Marcus R: Role of exercise in preventing and treating osteoporosis. Rheum Dis Clin North Am 2001;27:131–141.

32 Benardot D, Schwarz M, Heller DW: Nutrient intake in young, highly competitive gymnasts. J Am Diet Assoc 1989;89:401–403.

33 Lindholm C, Hagenfeldt K, Ringertz H: Bone mineral content of young female former gymnasts. Acta Paediatr 1995;84:1109–1112.

34 Robinson TL, Snow Harter C, Taafe DR, Gillis D, Shaw J, Marcus R: Gymnasts exhibit higher bone mass than runners despite similar prevalence of amenorrhea and oligomenorrhea. J Bone Miner Res 1995;10:26–35.

35 Kirchner EM, Lewis RD, O'Connor PJ: Effect of past gymnastics participation on adult bone mass. J Appl Physiol 1996;80:226–232.

36 Zanker CL, Osborne C, Cooke CB, Oldroyd B, Truscott JG: Bone density, body composition and menstrual history of sedentary female former gymnasts aged 20–32 years. Osteoporos Int 2004;15:87–92.

37 Snow CM, Rosen CJ, Robinson TL: Serum IGF-1 is higher in gymnasts than runners and predicts bone and lean mass. Med Sci Sports Exerc 2000;32:1902–1907.

38   Proctor KL, Adams WC, Shaffrath JD, Van Loan MD: Upper-limb bone mineral density of female collegiate gymnasts versus controls. Med Sci Sports Exerc 2002;34:1830–1835.

39   Helge EW, Kanstrup IL: Bone density in female elite gymnasts: impact of muscle strength and sex hormones. Med Sci Sports Exerc 2002;34:174–180.

40   Hassager C, Colwell A, Assiri AMA, Eastell R, Russell RG, Christiansen C: Effect of menopause and hormone replacement therapy on urinary excretion of pyridinium cross-links: a longitudinal and cross-sectional study. Clin Endocrinol 1992;37:45–50.

41   Turner RT, Riggs BL, Spelsberg TC: Skeletal effects of estrogen. Endocr Rev 1994;15:275–299.

42   Klibanski A, Biller BMK, Schoenfeld DA, Herzog DB, Saxe VC: The effects of estrogen administration on trabecular bone loss in young women with anorexia nervosa. J Clin Endocrinol Metab 1995;80:898–904.

43   Golden NH, Lanzkowsky HL, Scebendach CJ, Palestro CJ, Jacobson MS, Shenker IR: The effect of estrogen-progestin treatment on bone mineral density in anorexia nervosa. J Pediatr Adolesc Gynecol 2002;15:135–143.

44   Grinspoon S, Thomas L, Miller KK, Herzog DB, Klibanski A: Effects of recombinant human IGF-1 and oral contraceptive administration on bone density in anorexia nervosa. J Clin Endocrinol Metab 2002;87:2883–2891.

45   Munoz MT, Morande G, Garcia-Centenera JA, Hervas F, Pozo J, Argente J: The effects of estrogen administration on bone mineral density in adolescents with anorexia nervosa. J Clin Endocrinol Metab 2002;146:45–50.

46   Zanker CL, Swaine IL: The relationship between serum oestradiol concentration and energy balance in young women distance runners. Int J Sports Med 1998;19:104–108.

47   Grinspoon S, Baum H, Lee K, Anderson D, Herzog D, Klibanski A: Effects of short-term recombinant human insulin-like growth factor 1 administration on bone turnover in osteopenic women with anorexia nervosa. J Clin Endocrinol Metab 1996;81:3864–3870.

48   Hotta M, Shibasaki T, Sato K, Demura H: The importance of body weight history in the occurrence and recovery of osteoporosis in patients with anorexia nervosa: evaluation by dual X-ray absorptiometry and bone metabolic markers. Eur J Endocrinol 1998;139:276–283.

49   Hotta M, Fukuda I, Sato K, Hizuka N, Shibasaki T, Takano K: The relationship between bone turnover and body weight, serum IGF-1 and serum IGFBP levels in patients with anorexia nervosa. J Clin Endocrinol Metab 2000;85:200–206.

50   Kreipe RE, Hicks DG, Rosier RN, Puzas JE: Preliminary findings on the effects of sex hormones on bone metabolism in anorexia nervosa. J Adolesc Health 1993;14:319–324.

51   Heer M, Mika MC, Grzella I, Drummer C, Herpertz-Dahlmann B: Changes in bone turnover in patients with anorexia nervosa during eleven weeks of inpatient dietary treatment. Clin Chem 2002;48:754–760.

52   Heer M, Mika C, Grzella I, Heussen N, Herpertz-Dahlmann B: Bone turnover during inpatient nutrition therapy and outpatient follow-up in patients with anorexia nervosa compared with that in healthy control subjects. Am J Clin Nutr 2004;80:774–781.

53   Bachrach LK, Katzman DK, Litt IF, Guido D, Marcus R: Recovery from osteopenia in adolescent girls with anorexia nervosa. J Clin Endocrinol Metab 1991;72:602–606.

54   Miller KK, Lee EE, Lawson EA, Misra M, Minihan J, Grinspoon SK, Gleysteen S, Mickley D, Herzog D, Klibanski A: Determinants of skeletal loss and recovery in anorexia nervosa. J Clin Endocrinol Metab 2006;91:2931–2937.

55   Biller BMK, Saxe V, Herzog DB, Rosenthal DI, Holsman S, Klibanski A: Mechanisms of osteoporosis in adult and adolescent women with anorexia nervosa. J Clin Endocrinol Metab 1989;68: 548–554.

56   Misra M, Aggarwal A, Miller K, Almazan C, Worley M, Soyka L, Herzog D, Klibanski A: Effects of anorexia nervosa on clinical, hematologic, biochemical and bone density parameters in community dwelling adolescent girls. Pediatrics 2004;114:1574–1583.

57   Soyka LA, Grinspoon S, Levitsky LL, Herzog DB, Klibanski A: The effects of anorexia nervosa on bone metabolism in female adolescents. J Clin Endocrinol Metab 1999;84:4489–4496.

58   Serafinowicz E, Wasikowa R, Iwanicka Z, Jedrzejuk D: Bone metabolism in adolescent girls with short course of anorexia nervosa. Endokrynol Diabetol Chor Przemiany Materii Weiku Rozw 2003;9:67–71.

59 Soyka LA, Misra M, Frenchman A, Miller KK, Grinspoon S, Schoenfeld DA, Klibanski A: Abnormal bone mineral accrual in adolescent girls with anorexia nervosa. J Clin Endocrinol Metab 2002;87:4177–4185.

60 Grinspoon S, Thomas E, Pitts S, Gross E, Mikley D, Miller KK, Herzog DB, Klibanski A: Prevalence and predictive factors for regional osteopenia in women with anorexia nervosa. Ann Intern Med 2002;133:790–794.

61 Seeman E, Karlsson MK, Duan Y: On exposure to anorexia nervosa the temporal variation in axial and appendicular skeletal development predisposes to site-specific deficits in bone size and density: a cross-sectional study. J Bone Miner Res 2000;15:2259–2265.

62 Bass SL, Saxon L, Corral AM, Rodda CP, Strauss BJ, Reidpath D, Clarke C: Near normalisation of lumbar spine bone density in young women with osteopenia recovered from adolescent onset anorexia nervosa: a longitudinal study. J Pediatr Endocrinol Metab 2005;18:897–907.

63 Grinspoon SK, Baum HB, Peterson A, Coggins C, Klibanski A: Effects of short-term recombinant human insulin-like growth factor-1 administration on bone turnover during short-term fasting. J Clin Endocrinol Metab 1995;96:900–906.

64 Thissen JP, Ketelslegers JM, Underwood LE: Nutritional regulation of the insulin-like growth factors. Endocr Rev 1994;15:80–101.

65 Ammann P, Laib A, Bonjour JP, Meyer JM, Ruegsegger P, Rizzoli R: Dietary essential amino acid supplements increase bone strength by influencing bone mass and bone microarchitecture in ovariectomized adult rats fed an isocaloric low-protein diet. J Bone Miner Res 2002;17: 1264–1272.

66 Topaloglu AK, Yildizdas D, Yilmaz HL, Mungan NO, Yuksel B, Ozer G: Bone calcium changes during diabetic ketoacidosis: a comparison with lactic acidosis due to volume depletion. Bone 2005;37:122–127.

67 Musey VC, Goldstein S, Farmer PK, Moore PB, Phillips LS: Differential regulation of IGF-1 and IGF-binding protein-1 by dietary composition in humans. Am J Med Sci 1993;5:131–138.

68 Counts DR, Gwirtsman H, Carlsson LMS, Lesem M, Cutler G: The effects of anorexia nervosa and refeeding on growth hormone-binding protein, the insulin-like growth factors (IGFs) and the IGF-binding proteins. J Clin Endocrinol Metab 1992;75:762–766.

69 Argente J, Caballo JN, Barrios V, Munoz M, Pozo J, Chowen J, Morande G, Hernandez M: Multiple endocrine abnormalities of the growth hormone and insulin-like growth factor axis in patients with anorexia nervosa: effect of short- and long-term weight recuperation. J Clin Endocrinol Metab 1997;82:2084–2092.

70 Snow CM, Rosen CJ, Robinson TL: Serum IGF-1 is higher in gymnasts than runners and predicts bone and lean mass. Med Sci Sports Exerc 2000;32:1902–1907.

71 Zanker CL, Swaine IL: Responses of bone turnover markers to repeated endurance running under conditions of energy balance or energy restriction. Eur J Appl Physiol 2000;83:434–440.

72 Ihle R, Loucks AB: Dose response relations between energy availability and bone turnover in young, exercising women. J Bone Miner Res 2004;19:1231–1240.

73 Laughlin GA, Yen SSC: Hypoleptinemia in women athletes: absence of a diurnal rhythm with amenorrhea. J Clin Endocrinol Metab 1997;82:318–321.

74 Thong FS, Graham TE: Leptin and reproduction: is it a critical link between adipose tissue, nutrition and reproduction? Can J Appl Physiol 1999;24:317–336.

75 Thomas T, Gori F, Khosla S, Jensen MD, Burguera JB, Riggs BL: Leptin acts on human marrow stromal cells to enhance differentiation to osteoblasts and to inhibit differentiation to adipocytes. Endocrinology 1999;140:1630–1638.

76 Holloway WR, Collier FM, Aitkin CJ, Myers DE, Hodge JM, Malakellis M, Gough TJ, Collier GR, Nicholson GC: Leptin inhibits osteoclast generation. J Bone Miner Res 2002;17:200–209.

77 Kartensky G: Leptin controls bone formation through a hypothalamic relay. Recent Prog Horm Res 2001;56:401–415.

78 Welt CK, Chan JL, Bullen J, Murphy R, Smith P, DePaoli AM, Karalis A, Mantzoros CS: Recombinant human leptin in women with hypothalamic amenorrhea. N Engl J Med 2004;351: 987–997.

79 Bilanin JE, Blanchard MS, Russek-Cohen E: Lower vertebral bone density in male long distance runners. Med Sci Sports Exerc 1989;2:66–70.

80 Hetland ML, Haarbo J, Christiansen C: Low bone mass and high bone turnover in male long-distance runners. J Clin Endocrinol Metab 1993;77:770–775.
81 MacDougall JD, Webber CE, Martin J, Ormerod S, Chesley A, Younglai EV, Gordon CL, Blimkie CJR: Relationship among running mileage, bone density, and serum testosterone in male runners. J Appl Physiol 1992;73:1165–1170.
82 Stewart AD, Hannan J: Total and regional bone density in male runners, cyclists and controls. Med Sci Sports Exerc 2000;32:1373–1377.
83 Nichols JF, Palmer JE, Levy SS: Low bone mineral density in highly trained male master cyclists. Osteoporos Int 2003;14:644–649.
84 Daly RM, Rich PA, Klein R: Hormonal responses to physical training in high-level peripubertal male gymnasts. Eur J Appl Physiol Occup Physiol 1998;79:74–81.
85 Daly RM, Rich PA, Klein R, Bass SL: Short stature in competitive prepubertal and early pubertal male gymnasts: the result of selection bias or intense training? J Pediatr 2000;137:510–516.
86 Zanker CL, Swaine IL: The relationship between bone turnover, oestradiol and energy balance in women distance runners. Br J Sports Med 1998;32:167–171.

Dr. Cathy L. Zanker
Carnegie Research Institute
Carnegie Faculty of Sport and Education
Leeds Metropolitan University
Headingley Campus
Leeds, LS6 3QS (UK)
Tel. +44 113 283 2600, Fax +44 113 283 7575, E-Mail c.zanker@leedsmet.ac.uk

Daly R, Petit M (eds): Optimizing Bone Mass and Strength. The Role of Physical Activity and
Nutrition during Growth. Med Sport Sci. Basel, Karger, 2007, vol 51, pp 102–120

....

Risk Factors for Fractures in Normally Active Children and Adolescents

Ailsa Goulding

Department of Medical and Surgical Sciences, University of Otago,
Dunedin, New Zealand

Abstract

Although many children sustain at least one fracture during growth, the majority do
not, suggesting it is not the norm for healthy children to break their bones. Most childhood
fractures occur during play and sport and result from mild or moderate, rather than severe
trauma. The majority of fractures (86.4%) are treated solely in outpatient clinics. Furthermore,
there is evidence that 66% of all fractures during growth occur in children and adolescents
who fracture on more than one occasion, suggesting certain children may be predisposed to
fracture. These individuals frequently fracture first at a young age (<5 years), and any previous history of fracture increases the risk of further fractures 2- to 3-fold. While rates of fracture vary considerably with age, sex and maturation, they peak in early puberty when rates of
bone turnover are high but bone mineral accrual lags behind gains in height and weight.
Fractures are also common in children with endocrine dysfunction, chronic illnesses or
genetic disorders that affect bone metabolism and muscle mass, and/or require the use of
medications that influence bone metabolism. A number of risk factors have been identified
which may predispose children and adolescents to fracture. For instance, bone mineral content, bone size and bone accrual are all lower in apparently healthy children and adolescents
with fractures, and low bone mineral density is a predictor of new fracture. There is also evidence that genetic factors, poor nutrition (including an inadequate intake of dietary calcium,
milk avoidance and excessive consumption of carbonated beverages), lack of weight-bearing
physical activity, obesity and high exposure to trauma may influence fracture risks in the
general pediatric population.

Copyright © 2007 S. Karger AG, Basel

In the absence of chronic disease, osteoporotic fractures are rare in children and adolescents. However, fractures from falls are relatively common in
otherwise healthy children and adolescents, and are an important cause of pain
and morbidity in this age group. Fractures are the leading cause of admission to

hospital following injury. In a 10-year nationwide New Zealand survey of all hospital admissions for injury in children aged 0–14 years, 38.2% of the 106,666 admissions were due to fracture [1]. However, inpatient cases represent merely the tip of the iceberg, as only the more serious pediatric fracture cases require hospital admission [2, 3]. For instance, in a New Zealand study only 13.4% of children with confirmed fractures were admitted to hospital, with 86.6% receiving outpatient care [4]. Total treatment of childhood fractures (inpatient plus outpatient care) consumes a great deal of orthopedic, radiological, general practitioner and nursing time. Consequently, lowering fracture rates would improve child health and have considerable economic benefits. For this reason, there is increasing interest in the assessment and management of pediatric bone health and in identifying predictors of childhood fracture [5–10]. This chapter provides an overview of the epidemiology, risk factors, and strategies for the prevention of fractures in children and adolescents. The focus is primarily on otherwise healthy children and adolescents, rather than those with chronic disease or clinical conditions known to affect bone metabolism (e.g. osteogenesis imperfecta, rickets).

Epidemiology of Fractures during Growth

Evolutionary forces have ensured that all mammalian species grow bone which is suitable to meet the demands usually placed upon the skeleton [11]. Children fall frequently so it is important that their bones do not break during normal activities, play or sport. So what proportion of the pediatric population experiences any fracture? Landin [12], who conducted seminal studies on the epidemiology of childhood fractures in Sweden, calculated that by the age of 16 years the accumulated risks of having at least one fracture were 27% in girls and 42% in boys. In a birth cohort population of over 1,000 New Zealand children born in 1972–1973, Jones et al. [13] reported that 60.9% of girls and 49.3% of boys had never broken any bone between birth and 18 years. Stress fractures, which result from overuse and repetitive loading, are also uncommon in the general pediatric population, though they may affect young elite athletes [14, 15]. In one survey, only 2.7% of 5,461 American girls aged 11–17 years had any history of stress fractures [16].

Fracture Patterns Differ from Those of Adults
Children are not simply miniature adults and their fracture patterns differ from those of older adults. For instance, three quarters of childhood fractures affect the upper limbs [4] with the distal forearm being the most common site of fracture (25–30% of all fractures) [12, 13]. This is a fragility fracture, generally

resulting from modest trauma. Forearm fractures peak in early to mid puberty (10–12 years in girls and 13–15 years in boys) [17], which coincides with the period of rapid skeletal growth and an increased demand of newly formed bone for minerals [18, 19], reshaping of the radial metaphysis [20], elevated bone turnover [21], and an increase in growth-regulating hormones. At this time, bone mineral accrual is most discordant with gains in body weight and height [22]: gains in total body and regional bone mineral accrual lag behind increases in both height and weight, resulting in a transient deficit in bone mass relative to longitudinal growth [23]. Fortunately, once bone mass reaches adult values, distal forearm fracture rates fall sharply [11]. They remain low in men, who maintain adequate bone mass at this site, but rise in older women, who lose bone mineral at the forearm when estrogen levels decline [24]. Other frequent sites of childhood fracture include the humerus (11%), hands (20%), and fingers, foot bones and clavicle [25]. Lower limb fractures occur less often, and hip fractures are rare, as are fractures of the ribs and vertebrae. Fractures at these sites in children are typically associated with severe trauma, disease, use of bone-thinning medications or child abuse [26].

Fracture Rates Vary with Age and Sex

All populations exhibit a biphasic pattern of fracture throughout life, with rates peaking during adolescence and old age and remaining lower in mid adulthood [27]. During growth, fracture patterns vary with age, gender and pubertal maturation [25]. For example, fractures of the humerus peak at a younger age than those of the radius, while fractures of the hand bones have a substantially higher prevalence in teenagers [28]. Boys typically experience more fractures than girls, despite having larger and stronger skeletons. This is probably because males are exposed to more high-risk activities leading to severe trauma and have higher peak growth rates than females [28]. Presumably a difference in the rate and timing of bone mineral accretion at different skeletal regions, and age-related changes in the way children fall and protect their limbs when striking the ground or playing sports may also, at least partially, account for age-related variations in fractures. Furthermore, there is evidence that children with delayed bone maturation for chronological age have an increased risk of fracture, which is likely to be related to delayed mineral accrual and reduced strength [29].

A Few Children Sustain Most of the Fractures

Few accidents induce fractures at multiple skeletal sites. Only 1.7% of 3,350 children with limb fractures had broken more than one bone from the same accident [2]. However, more children break bones on a number of different occasions. In a study conducted in New Zealand children and adolescents, only one third of the total fracture burden between birth and age 18 years was borne by individuals who experience a single fracture [30]. In contrast, two thirds of all the fractures occur in a smaller subset of apparently healthy children who repeatedly fracture a bone (15.8% of girls and 23.4% of boys in this birth cohort sample). These findings reinforce the view that it is not the norm for healthy children to fracture during growth, and indicate that children who fracture bones repeatedly do so because of some underlying risk factors for fracture.

Trauma Precipitates Fracture

In the absence of clinical disease (such as osteogenesis imperfecta), few children break bones spontaneously as may occur in adults with severe osteoporosis, and typically some force or high-energy trauma precipitates each fracture. Most childhood fractures are incurred during normal play and sport. The majority are associated with only minimal trauma (falls from less than standing height) or moderate trauma (falls from >1 m or higher-velocity accidents) and less than 10% of all childhood fractures involve major trauma, such as traffic accidents or falls from >3 m [12]. However, fractures associated with high-velocity impact or falls from greater heights tend to be more serious. In 1,405 playground falls, children falling from a height were more likely to suffer fractures requiring reduction (realignment) than those falling from less than standing height [OR, 3.91 (95% CI 2.76–5.54)] [3]. In addition, increasing body mass substantially increases the impact of a fall, so that obese children place greater force on the bone during a fall [11, 31], which may help to explain the higher fracture risks of overweight children [32, 33].

Childhood Fractures Are Becoming More Common

Although it is not the norm to fracture, fracture rates in children and adolescents are currently increasing, particularly at the forearm. In the United States, rates increased by 56% in girls and 32% in boys between 1969–1999 [34]. Between 1986–1995, fracture rates rose by 14% in Japan [35] and 45% in Australia [36], with similar rises also reported in France [37]. The magnitude and rapidity of these increases suggest that environmental changes, rather than genetic factors or underlying disease(s), may be responsible. In the following section, risk factors found to be associated with fractures in children and adolescents will be reviewed.

Risk Factors for Fracture during Growth

Risk factors for childhood fractures can be classified as genetic, intrinsic, or environmental. They could reflect greater skeletal fragility from poor nutrition,

Table 1. Factors contributing to increased fracture risks during growth

Rapid changes in the shape and microarchitecture of the bones
High osteoclastic and osteoblastic cellular activity
History of previous fracture, particularly at a young age
History of prolonged milk avoidance
Small or narrow bones
Low bone mineral content
Mismatch of body weight and height to bone mineral accrual
Overweight or obesity (heavy falls and insufficient adaptive skeletal changes)
Insufficient intermittent weight-bearing activity to optimize bone development
Inadequate outdoor activity to safeguard vitamin D status
Nutrition inadequate to cater for the high demands of new bone
Unhealthy beverage choices (carbonated soft drink)
High intakes of foods augmenting urinary calcium losses (salt, caffeine)
High-risk-taking behavior
Participation in dangerous activities and/or extreme sports
Frequent falls or exposure to high-velocity impacts (contact and ball sports)
Hypogonadism (primary or secondary)
Behavior jeopardizing estrogen status (anorexia or athletic amenorrhea)
Smoking cigarettes, taking excessive alcohol, watching too much TV

insufficient load bearing or hormonal dysfunction. Alternatively, they could be due to more frequent participation in behavior which places bones at higher risk of breaking [38]. In most studies, only a minority of children presenting with fractures have been diagnosed with serious diseases or are being treated with medications or radiotherapy that lead to reduced bone mineral accrual and skeletal fragility. Unfortunately, although circumstances of fracture are generally recorded after the occurrence of a fracture, little attention has been devoted to the potential influence of modifiable factors, such as poor nutrition, inadequate exercise, impaired musculoskeletal coordination or low bone mass (osteopenia), in promoting fracture. Some of the key risk factors associated with fractures during childhood and adolescence are listed in table 1 and are discussed below. These include: age at first fracture, low bone mass, size and strength, musculoskeletal weakness, along with hormonal, genetic and environmental factors.

Children with Repeated Fractures Usually
Fracture First at a Young Age

It seems likely that children with inherently weak skeletons will fracture at a young age and then continue to fracture [4, 30, 33]. As in adults, children who sustain a first fracture are at substantially increased risk of further fracture. For instance, hazard ratios for sustaining a further fracture were 1.90 (95% CI 1.50–2.49) after a first fracture and 3.04 (95% CI 2.23–4.15) after a second fracture [30]. Interestingly, although most fractures (66%) occur during adolescence, the majority of individuals who experience repeated fractures have their first fracture at a younger age. For instance, in the New Zealand birth cohort population study only 16.8% of the children with multiple fractures experienced their first fracture during adolescence while 83.2% sustained their first fracture before they reached their teens. Moreover, half the children who had a fracture before the age of 13 years suffered an additional fracture, whereas only one in five of those who had experienced their first fracture as teenagers had further fractures. This suggests that fracture events during adolescence are likely due to simple accidents or represent a transient reduction in bone mass which soon normalizes. In contrast, children who fracture at a young age may have some underlying bone disease or risk factors that need to be evaluated carefully so that appropriate measures can be put into place to optimize their bone health to reduce their risk of further fractures.

Children Who Fracture Have Lower Bone Mass

Low areal bone mineral density (aBMD) is a major risk factor for fracture in adults [39] and it would seem plausible that low aBMD should also increase pediatric fracture risk. A number of different groups using single photon absorptiometry [40], dual-energy X-ray absorptiometry [41–46], computed tomography [47], peripheral quantitative computed tomography [48, 49], and ultrasound [50, 51] have confirmed that aBMD, bone mineral content (BMC), bone quality and sometimes bone size [47] are reduced in children and adolescents with fractures compared to fracture-free controls. There is also evidence that children with long narrow bones are more liable to fracture than those having shorter, broader bones [47]. Importantly, reductions in total body aBMD were predictive of new fracture in a 4-year prospective study of 170 girls, with the risk approximately doubling for each standard deviation decrease in aBMD at baseline [32]. In the same study, previous fractures, low aBMD and high body weight were identified as independent factors associated with an increased risk of sustaining new fractures, with the hazard ratios rising to between 10 and 13 in children having more than one of these risk factors in combination [32]. Another important cohort study of 125 Swiss girls followed for 8.5 years reported that bone mineral accrual at multiple sites was lower at maturity in the 42 girls who fractured during the study, compared with those who had no fractures [46]. The authors suggested that childhood fractures may be a marker of low peak bone mass acquisition and persistent skeletal fragility. Reductions in bone mass have also been documented in many pediatric fracture patients with poor nutrition, endocrine disorders, congenital conditions adversely affecting bone development, or chronic disease, as well as in healthy children who have broken bones after modest trauma.

Musculoskeletal Weakness

Children with chronic diseases and genetic disorders associated with musculoskeletal weakness, including low muscle mass and strength, generally have low aBMD and are liable to fracture long bones with minimal trauma. This pattern is seen in Duchenne's muscular dystrophy [52, 53], cystic fibrosis [54], cerebral palsy [55], and sickle cell disease [56]. Fractures of the lower extremities are more common in such populations, and can lead to permanent loss of ambulation [57]. However, it appears that the severity of the disease influences fracture risk; rates do not seem to be elevated in less severe cases. For instance, fracture rates in children with mild cystic fibrosis did not differ from those observed in healthy controls [hazard ratio 0.96 (95% CI 0.68–1.30)] [58].

Gait disorders, impaired motor skills, poor balance and postural instability also act to increase falls in children, and may thus precipitate fracture. Adults with epilepsy have two to six times the fracture risk of the general population [59]. Their propensity to fracture may be related to seizures, frequent unprotected falls or use of antiepileptic medications [59]. Data in children with epilepsy are scarce, though restrictions in physical activity, use of anticonvulsant medications and a tendency to suffer awkward falls probably increase their risk of fractures [60].

High Adiposity

Although obesity does stimulate adaptive increases in bone mass and size, BMC in relation to body weight is reduced in obese children [61, 62]. High adiposity seems to be an important risk factor for forearm fractures [32]. In large samples of girls and boys with forearm fractures, total body percentage fat was increased [49] and overweight and obesity were overrepresented in the fracture cases [33, 41, 42]. In many obese adolescents, the mismatch in the gain in bone mass relative to body weight is exaggerated because there is a greater gain in fat mass compared to lean mass. Since bone adapts to muscle forces rather than to static loads imposed by extra fat mass [63], this may put overweight children at an increased risk of fracture. High adiposity associated with low levels of growth hormone [64], or high levels of corticosteroids [65] may also elevate fracture risks in children, particularly when muscle mass is decreased, though this is not always seen [66].

Heavy and obese children have greater rates of injury than those of normal weight. In a Belgian study of over 2,000 children aged 9–17 years, the rate of injury requiring treatment by a health professional was higher in overweight children (BMI values >85th percentile) than among those of healthy weight

[OR, 1.36 (95% CI 1.07–1.76)], though risks of severe injury requiring hospital admission did not achieve significance [OR, 1.19 (95% CI 0.72–1.95)] [67]. Inactivity and indolence favor fat gain, and many obese children habitually avoid physical activity, which may impair their musculoskeletal development and coordination. For instance, obese children have been shown to have poor gross balance compared to those of normal weight, possibly because they have more inert fat mass to manage relative to their muscle mass, as posturography suggests visual perception and fine motor skills are similar in obese and nonobese individuals [68].

Medications with Toxic Actions on Bone

Many young children with asthma, arthritis, malabsorption syndromes, cancer and organ transplantation have low bone mass. This is probably due to the combined adverse effects of underlying pediatric illness, disturbances in the control of osteoclastic activity via the osteoprotegerin/RANK ligand cascade, the bone-thinning actions of medications and radiotherapy, as well as hypogonadism, suboptimal nutrition (particularly protein, vitamin D and calcium), reduced physical activity and muscle weakness [7]. After heart, renal or marrow transplantation, there is evidence that children have reduced aBMD and even spinal fractures [69]. Children treated with immunosuppressive therapy and chemotherapy for malignancies such as leukemia also develop striking osteopenia, and are prone to develop fractures [70]. Corticosteroids are widely used in sick children and may contribute to fractures. In 383,310 British children aged 4–17 years, fracture risk was increased by high doses of oral corticosteroids [OR, 1.32 (95% CI 1.03–1.69)] [71]. However, a dose-dependent increase in fracture risk in children using inhaled corticosteroids disappeared after adjustment for asthma severity, suggesting that disease severity, rather than inhaled steroid use, explains much of the increased risks of fracture in asthmatic children [72]. Vitamin K deficiency has adverse effects on bone health and chronic use of warfarin, a vitamin K antagonist, by children with congenital heart disease was found to be associated with reduced aBMD [73]. Though fracture rates in such pediatric populations have not been assessed, adult population-based data have provided evidence that the use of anticoagulants for 12 months or more was associated with substantial increases in standardized incidence rates (SIR) for both vertebral [SIR, 5.3 (95% CI 3.4–8.0)] and rib fractures [SIR, 3.4 (95% CI 1.8–5.7)] [74].

Genetic Factors

Many pediatric fracture cases report a family history of fractures, suggesting inherited factors or a common lifestyle may contribute to their propensity to fracture. A survey of 1,246 teenagers found 29.2% of those without fractures,

38.9% of those with a single fracture and 51.6% of those with multiple fractures had a positive family history of fracture [75]. The classic example of an inherited genetic factor that elevates fracture risk is osteogenesis imperfecta, where bone collagen defects explain bone weakness and fragility [76]. Milk avoidance, though often familial, is not always due to an inherited intolerance to lactose or milk proteins: fracture risks can be due to common family nutritional risk factors such as calcium and protein deprivation, rather than to inherited bone weakness [77]. However, given the many growth factors which can influence bone metabolism, it seems likely that future genetic studies will be fruitful in improving our understanding of fracture epidemiology, particularly in children who sustain repeated fractures [9].

Intrauterine Factors

Many adult diseases are influenced by fetal development and some consider poor intrauterine and early growth may contribute to fracture risk [78]. Very-low-birth-weight infants have light, poorly mineralized skeletons, and are prone to fracture [79]. Maternal smoking, vitamin D deficiency, prematurity and low birth weight are associated with lower adult bone mass and higher fracture rates later in life. This suggests that the adverse effects of early nutrition and programming of endocrine axes on bone health may be long-lasting [80]. Thus, optimization of nutrition for both mother and baby would appear to be an important strategy to lower subsequent fracture risk.

Nutritional Factors

It seems possible that even transient periods of illness and hormonal dysfunction due to nutritional insufficiency during critical periods of growth could result in persisting site-specific deficits in bone mass which would make these people vulnerable to fracture [22]. Adequate nutrition is very important to optimal skeletal health and it is vital that the diet provides all the essential minerals, energy, micronutrients and vitamins necessary for growth in bone length and mass. To date, there have been relatively few studies that have assessed the link between particular nutrients and fracture risk in children. There is some work to suggest that fetal malnutrition, milk avoidance, low intakes of dietary calcium, energy deprivation, and vitamin D insufficiency may increase fracture risk. In addition, excessive intakes of carbonated drinks have also been linked to fractures in children.

Inadequate Dietary Calcium

Insufficient intake of dietary calcium to meet the demands of rapid skeletal growth may limit bone development and increase fracture risk; there is also evidence that the non-weight-bearing radius is particularly susceptible to insufficient dietary calcium [33, 81]. Vitamin D insufficiency reduces the ability to absorb dietary calcium and severe deficits impair bone mineralization. Increasing obligatory calcium losses raises the dietary requirement for calcium: high intakes of salty foods, caffeine or sulfur-containing amino acids have all been linked to increased calcium losses. Although low maternal vitamin D status is associated with reduced bone density in children [78], no studies appear to have yet examined childhood fracture rates in relation to vitamin D insufficiency or hypercalciuria, or looked at the ability of calcium supplementation to reduce pediatric fractures.

Calorie Deprivation

Hypogonadism (both male and female) is associated with low bone mass. Girls who slim or exercise to excess often have low circulating estrogen levels. They have lower leptin levels and lower bone mass compared to girls with normal menstrual function [82–84]. Fractures and low aBMD are associated with low estrogen status in patients with athletic amenorrhea, anorexia nervosa and hyperprolactinemia. A nationwide survey of fracture risk in 942 Danish patients with eating disorders showed that their fracture risk was approximately doubled, compared to age- and gender-matched controls [incidence rate ratio, 1.98 (95% CI 1.60–2.44)] [85]. Moreover, risks remained elevated more than 10 years after diagnosis, suggesting skeletal damage associated with lack of estrogen during growth persists into adult life.

Beverage Choices

Cola and soft drinks provide excessive calories but few essential nutrients. Some also contain caffeine, which is hypercalciuric. There are concerns that high consumption of such drinks may lead to obesity and reductions in the intake of milk. Wyshak [86] first reported that children consuming large amounts of carbonated beverages had more fractures. Some studies [87], but not all [4], confirm this association. A weak inverse association between aBMD and carbonated drink consumption has been reported in girls but not boys [88], suggesting greater milk displacement in the girls [89].

Milk Avoidance

Milk is a rich source of nutrients essential for normal skeletal growth [90]. Several lines of evidence now support the view that chronic milk avoidance without compensatory dietary adjustments increases fracture risk in otherwise healthy children. Thus, young milk avoiders have shorter stature and smaller skeletons with lower bone mass than those who consume milk regularly [77, 91–96]. Furthermore, standardized rates of fracture were 2- to 3-fold higher in milk avoiders compared to milk drinkers of similar age and gender [90], with one in three experiencing a fracture before the age of 8 years. Such children seemed particularly prone to fracture their forearms and to suffer recurrent fractures [97]. Moreover, in a sample of 1,880 adults from the NHANES III study, women who drank milk less than once a week in childhood and adolescence had higher rates of osteoporotic fractures late in life than those who drank milk daily during growth [98]. This finding is consistent with the view that peak bone mass is reduced in young adults who avoided milk during growth [99]. Prolonged milk avoidance was more common in Polish teenagers with multiple fractures than in fracture-free controls (18.6 vs. 12.4%, p < 0.001) [75]. Adverse symptoms to milk, such as eczema, rhinitis and gastrointestinal discomfort and low milk consumption were more common than expected in a consecutive series of fracture cases under 13 years of age [4]. Adverse symptoms to milk were also overrepresented in children with multiple forearm fractures, with youngsters having a history of symptoms to milk showing reduced BMC in the ultradistal radius [33].

Cigarette Smoking

Cigarette smoking lowers bone mass and increases osteoporotic fracture risks in adults [100]. A meta-analysis of 512,399 adults reported the pooled relative risk for all fracture types in current smokers was 1.26 (95% CI 1.12–1.42) [101]. Cigarette smoking also seems detrimental to bone health during growth. In a birth cohort population of adolescents in New Zealand who smoked daily, the risk of fracture was significantly increased relative to those who never smoked [relative risk, 1.43 (95% CI 1.05–1.95)] [102].

Strategies for Preventing Fractures during Growth

Creating a Safe Play and Sport Environment

Improving the safety of sport is an important strategy to limit childhood and adolescent fractures since many sporting environments increase the risk of fracture. A review of 1,255 children aged 5–15 years treated in accident and emergency at a British hospital showed that a fifth (20.3%) of children seen because of injury during sport had suffered a fracture [103]. Two thirds of all sport-related emergency clinic visits occur in persons aged 5–24, with males having double the injury visits compared to females [104]. Most of these sport-related fractures result from falls. Consequently, it is important that playgrounds are safe, contact sports are well supervised and children participating in sports such as gymnastics are taught how to fall safely [38]. Appropriate protective gear should always be worn when participating in dangerous sports so as to limit risks of fracture [105, 106]. Clinical trials have shown this strategy can reduce fractures [107, 108].

Limiting Risk-Taking Behavior

Hyperactivity, impulsive behavior, poor perception of danger, or greater participation in high-risk activities may also increase the risk of fracture [109]. A population-based study of 20,025 British Columbians aged 19 years who were considered to have behavior disorders because they had been prescribed methylphenidate showed an increased odds ratio for hospital admission for fracture in comparison to more than a million controls never prescribed this drug [OR, 1.42 (95% CI 1.27–1.58)]. Ma et al. [110] evaluated risk-taking behavior in a population-based group of Tasmanian adolescents with upper limb fractures using a 5-item interview-administered questionnaire. They reported that high-risk-taking behavior was associated with fractures of the hand bones, which were mostly incurred playing sport [OR, 2.6 (95% CI 1.1–5.7)], but not with fractures of the upper arm or distal forearm where poor balance was more important.

Management of Low aBMD

Since low aBMD and reduced bone mineral accrual are important risk factors for fracture in children, measurements of bone mass may be helpful in evaluating the skeletal health of children presenting with recurrent fractures after minimal trauma, and those showing extreme osteopenia on plain X-ray. However, aBMD assessment should not be routinely recommended at the time of first fracture. Pediatric patients with recurrent fractures, or conditions associated with considerably elevated risks of fracture, such as those with osteogenesis imperfecta, and children using high-dose corticosteroids or under treatment for leukemia may warrant the use of bone-sparing therapies such as bisphosphonates. Bisphosphonate treatment elevates bone mass, lowers bone pain and reduces fractures in osteogenesis imperfecta [76, 111, 112]. However, the use of bisphosphonates should be reserved to specialist units with expertise in treating pediatric bone disorders since these agents linger in bone and the long-term consequences of therapy remain to be established [113]. Bisphosphonates should not be used in pregnancy as they cross the placenta [6].

General Strategies to Reduce Fractures during Growth

Healthy bones should not fracture with the stresses of normal play and sport. Although we will never prevent all accidents and some fractures will therefore be inevitable, we should strive to reduce fracture rates during childhood and adolescence. Table 2 summarizes some general strategies to help achieve this. In order to develop strong bones which do not fracture easily it is important to encourage children to attain their genetically potential peak bone mass during the first two decades of life. Maintaining good bone mass subsequently will also help to reduce osteoporotic fractures later in life. Throughout

Table 2. Strategies to lower risk of fracture in children and adolescents

Achieve maximal genetic peak bone mass
Maintain healthy body weight
Undertake daily weight-bearing exercise
Encourage regular sport and play in a safe environment
Consume a balanced diet that fully satisfies needs for protein and energy
Consume adequate dietary calcium
Maintain adequate vitamin D status
Do not overexercise or slim to the point of amenorrhea
Do not smoke cigarettes or drink alcohol in excess
Wear appropriate safety gear for dangerous sports

growth, children and adolescents need a balanced diet, regular weight-bearing physical activity and healthy endocrine development. They should aim to consume a diet meeting the recommended needs for essential nutrients and should maintain a healthy body weight, good muscle mass and adequate vitamin D status. They should develop a broad range of motor skills and coordination to improve balance and help prevent falls which may predispose to fractures.

Leisure activities should take place in a safe environment. Playground equipment should meet safety standards and young children should be supervised when playing. Adolescents should wear protective clothing when engaging in dangerous sports or activities (cycle helmets, knee and elbow pads, wrist guards when skateboarding or snowboarding, appropriate boots when skiing or skating, and protective hats when riding horses). Because children mature at different rates, only children and teenagers of similar body build should play competitive sports together.

Health care professionals should be particularly alert to safeguard bone health in calorie-conscious athletes and amenorrheic girls since excessive slimming and/or athletic behavior associated with estrogen deficiency is extremely damaging to the skeleton. Smoking cigarettes, and excessive intakes of caffeine, salt, alcohol or soft drinks can also be detrimental to bone health. Milk avoidance without compensatory nutritional changes, inadequate dietary intakes of calcium and protein, and vitamin D insufficiency are other important nutritional problems that are likely to increase fracture risk if they are prolonged. Monitoring the nutrition, physical activity and bone health of children having these problems is therefore particularly important.

Health professionals should also carefully review the skeletal health of every child presenting with a first fracture (table 3). Clear remedial advice to optimize bone health should then be provided for the children and their families to follow. Children who have syndromes known to be associated with fractures

Table 3. Useful checklist for every child or adolescent presenting with fracture

Fracture circumstances
How did the fracture happen? (slight or severe trauma)
Was fracture appropriate for circumstances? (consider possible abuse/bullying)
Has the child had any previous fractures?
If so, how many, which bones and at what age did the fractures occur?

Possible genetic factors
Is there any family history of fracture?
Was the child a premature baby?
Has the child any illnesses or inherited syndromes affecting bone?
Are there any signs of endocrine disorders?
Are any bone-thinning medications or treatments being given?

Anthropometry
Weigh and measure the child (calculate BMI)
Does the child have normal height and BMI for age?
Is he/she currently overweight or underweight?
Assess pubertal status (Tanner stage) and menstrual regularity

Physical activity
Does the child play sport and undertake sufficient regular weight-bearing activity?
Is exercise excessive for calorie intake?
Does he/she use appropriate safety gear for sports?
Is he/she well coordinated?

Nutrition
Is the child receiving balanced nutrition? (consider calories, vitamin D, calcium, protein,
    beverage choices, salt, caffeine)
Does he/she have any food allergies or any history of milk avoidance?

Behavior
Does he/she smoke cigarettes or drink alcohol on a regular basis?
Is he/she a high-risk taker?

or who utilize medications that induce bone loss need to be monitored once their condition has been diagnosed and *before they fracture.* Assessment of aBMD or BMC can be useful in such patients, but these measurements need to be interpreted by units experienced in managing pediatric bone health. Parents, families, friends, schools, coaches, general practitioners and the community all have an important role to play in improving bone health and lowering fracture rates of children and adolescents. To date, there have been no well-designed long-term intervention trials examining whether improved nutrition and physical activity can lower future fracture rates in children and adolescents. Given that fracture rates appear to be increasing in children, such trials would appear to be warranted.

References

1   Kypri K, Chalmers DJ, Langley JD, Wright CS: Child injury morbidity in New Zealand, 1987–1996. J Paediatr Child Health 2001;37:227–234.

2   Cheng JCY, Shen WY: Limb fracture pattern in different pediatric age groups: a study of 3,350 children. J Orthop Trauma 1993;7:15–22.

3   Fiissel D, Pattison G, Howard A: Severity of playground fractures: play equipment versus standing height falls. Inj Prev 2005;11:337–339.

4   Yeh F-J, Grant AM, Williams SM, Goulding A: Children who experience their first fracture at a young age have high rates of fracture. Osteoporos Int 2006;17:267–272.

5   Bachrach LK: Osteoporosis and measurement of bone mass in children and adolescents. Endocrinol Metab Clin North Am 2005;34:521–535.

6   Bianchi ML: How to manage osteoporosis in children. Best Pract Res Clin Rheumatol 2005;19: 991–1005.

7   Ward LM: Osteoporosis due to glucocorticoid use in children with chronic illness. Horm Res 2005;64:209–221.

8   Aris RM, Merkel PA, Bachrach LK, Burowitz DS, Boyle MP, Elkin SL, Guise TA, Hardin DS, Hawarth CS, Holick MF, Joseph PM, O'Brien K, Tullis E, Watts NB, White TB: Consensus statement: guide to bone health and disease in cystic fibrosis. J Clin Endocrinol Metab 2005;90: 1888–1896.

9   Tinkle BT, Wenstrup RJ: A genetic approach to fracture epidemiology in childhood. Am J Med Genet 2005;139C:38–54.

10 Gelfand IM, DiMeglio LA: Bone mineral accrual and low bone mass: a pediatric perspective. Rev Endocrinol Metab Disord 2005;6:281–289.

11 Currey JD: How well are bones designed to resist fracture? J Bone Min Res 2003;18:591–598.

12 Landin LA: Fracture patterns in children. Acta Orthop Scand Suppl 1983;54:1–109.

13 Jones IE, Williams SM, Dow N, Goulding A: How many children remain fracture-free during growth? A longitudinal study of children and adolescents participating in the Dunedin Multi-disciplinary Health and Development Study. Osteoporos Int 2002;13:990–995.

14 Ohta-Fukushima M, Mutoh Y, Takasugi S, Iwata H, Ishii S: Characteristics of stress fractures in young athletes under 20 years. J Sports Med Phys Fitness 2002;42:198–206.

15 Kang L, Belcher D, Hulstyn MJ: Stress fractures of the femoral shaft in women's college lacrosse: a report of seven cases and a review of the literature. Br J Sports Med 2005;39:902–906.

16 Loud KJ, Gordon CM, Micheli LJ, Field AE: Correlates of stress fractures among preadolescent and adolescent girls. Pediatrics 2005;115:e399–e406.

17 Blimkie CJR, Lefevre J, Beunen GP, Renson R, Dequeker J, Van Damme P: Fractures, physical activity, and growth velocity in adolescent Belgian boys. Med Sci Sports Exerc 1993;25: 801–808.

18 Matkovic V: Nutrition, genetics and skeletal development. J Am Coll Nutr 1996;15:556–569.

19 Magarey AM, Boulton TJC, Chatterton BE, Schultz C, Nordin BEC, Cockington RA: Bone growth from 11 to 17 years: relationship to growth, gender and changes with pubertal status including timing of menarche. Acta Paediatr 1999;88:139–146.

20 Rauch F, Neu C, Manz F, Schoenau E: The development of metaphyseal cortex – implications for distal radius fractures during growth. J Bone Min Res 2001;16:1547–1555.

21 Heaney RP, Weaver CM: Newer perspectives on calcium nutrition and bone quality. J Am Coll Nutr 2005;24:574S–581S.

22 Bass S, Delmas PD, Pearce G, Hendrich E, Tabensky A, Seeman E: The differing tempo of growth in bone size, mass, and density in girls is region-specific. J Clin Invest 1999;104:795–804.

23 Fournier PE, Rizzoli R, Slosman DO, Theintz G, Bonjour JP: Asynchrony between the rates of standing height gain and bone mass accumulation during puberty. Osteoporos Int 1997;7: 525–532.

24 Khosla S, Riggs BL, Atkinson EJ, Oberg AL, McDaniel LJ, Holets M, Peterson JM, Melton LJ: Effects of sex and age on bone microstructure at the ultradistal radius: a population-based noninvasive in vivo assessment. J Bone Miner Res 2006;21:124–131.

25 Cooper C, Dennison EM, Leufkens HGM, Bishop N, Van Staa TP: Epidemiology of childhood fractures in Britain: a study using the General Practice Research Database. J Bone Miner Res 2004;19:1976–1981.

26 Bulloch B, Schubert CJ, Brophy PD, Johnson N, Reed MH, Shapiro RA: Cause and clinical characteristics of rib fractures in infants. Pediatrics 2000;105:e48.

27 Alffram P-A, Bauer GCH: Epidemiology of fractures of the forearm: a biomechanical investigation of bone strength. J Bone Joint Surg Am 1962;44:105–114.

28 Vadivelu R, Dias JJ, Burke FD, Stanton J: Hand injuries in children. A prospective study. J Pediatr Orthop 2006;26:29–35.

29 Ma DQ, Jones G: Skeletal age deviation assessed by the Tanner-Whitehouse 2 method is associated with bone mass and fracture risk in children. Bone 2005;36:352–357.

30 Goulding A, Jones IE, Williams SM, Grant AM, Taylor RW, Manning PJ, Langley J: First fracture is associated with increased risk of new fractures during growth. J Pediatr 2005;146:286–288.

31 Davidson PL, Goulding A, Chalmers DJ: Biomechanical analysis of arm fracture in obese boys. J Paediatr Child Health 2003;39:657–664.

32 Goulding A, Jones IE, Taylor RW, Manning PJ, Williams SM: More broken bones: a 4-year double cohort study of young girls with and without distal forearm fractures. J Bone Miner Res 2000;15: 2011–2018.

33 Goulding A, Grant AM, Williams SM: Bone and body composition of children and adolescents with repeated forearm fractures. J Bone Miner Res 2005;20:2090–2096.

34 Khosla S, Melton LJ, Dekutoski MB, Achenbach SJ, Oberg AL, Riggs BL: Incidence of childhood distal forearm fractures over 30 years. A population-based study. JAMA 2003;290:1479–1485.

35 Hagino H, Yamamoto K, Ohshiro H, Nose T: Increasing incidence of distal radius fractures in Japanese children and adolescents. J Orthop Sci 2000;5:356–360.

36 Sherker S, Ozanne-Smith J: Are current playground safety standards adequate for preventing arm fractures? Med J Aust 2004;180:562–565.

37 Lautman S, Bergerault F, Bonnard C, Laumonier F, Bronfen C, Mallet JF, Rogez JM, Chappuis M, Bracq H, Abuamara S, Lechevallier J: Epidemiological survey of wrist fractures in children. Rev Chir Orthop Reparatrice Appar Mot 2003;89:399–403.

38 Shields BJ, Smith GA: Cheerleading-related injuries to children 5 to 18 years of age: United States 1990–2002. Pediatrics 2006;129:122–129.

39 Johnell O, Kanis JA, Oden A, Johansson H, DeLaet C, Delmas P, Eisman JA, Fujiwara S, Kroger H, Mellstrom D, Meunier PJ, Melton LJ, O'Neill T, Pols H, Reeve J, Silman A, Tenenhouse A: Predictive value of BMD for hip and other fractures. J Bone Miner Res 2005;20:1185–1194.

40 Landin L, Nilsson BE: Bone mineral content in children with fractures. Clin Orthop 1983;178:292–296.

41 Goulding A, Cannan R, Williams SM, Gold EJ, Taylor RW, Lewis-Barned NJ: Bone mineral density in girls with forearm fractures. J Bone Miner Res 1998;13:143–148.

42 Goulding A, Jones IE, Taylor RW, Manning PJ, Williams SM: Bone mineral density and body composition in boys with distal forearm fractures: a dual-energy X-ray absorptiometry study. J Pediatr 2001;139:509–515.

43 Ma DQ, Jones G: The association between bone mineral density, metacarpal morphometry, and upper limb fractures in children: a population-based case-control study. J Clin Endocrinol Metab 2003;88:1486–1491.

44 Crabtree NJ, Kibirige MS, Fordham JN, Banks LM, Muntoni F, Chinn CM, Boivin CM, Shaw NJ: The relationship between lean mass and bone mineral content in paediatric health and disease. Bone 2004;35:965–972.

45 Horlick M, Wang J, Pierson RN, Thornton JC: Prediction models for evaluation of total-body bone mass with dual-energy X-ray absorptiometry among children and adolescents. Pediatrics 2004;114: e337–e345.

46 Ferrari SL, Chevalley T, Bonjour J-P, Rizzoli R: Childhood fractures are associated with decreased bone mass gain during puberty: an early marker of persistent bone fragility? J Bone Miner Res 2006;21:501–507.

47 Skaggs DL, Loro ML, Pitukcheewanont P, Tolo V, Gilsanz V: Increased body weight and decreased radial cross-sectional dimensions in girls with forearm fractures. J Bone Miner Res 2001;16: 1337–1342.

48 Landoll JD, Mobley SL, Ha E, Badenhop-Stevens NE, Hangartner TN, Matkovic V: Children with bone fragility fractures have reduced volumetric bone mineral density of the radius. J Bone Miner Res 2004;19:S87.

49 Mobley SL, Ha E, Landoll JD, Badenhop-Stevens NE, Clairmont A, Goel P, Matkovic V: Children with bone fragility fractures have reduced bone mineral areal density at the forearm and hip and higher percent body fat. J Bone Miner Res 2005;(suppl 1):S34.

50 Fielding KT, Nix DA, Bachrach LK: Comparison of calcaneus ultrasound and dual X-ray absorptiometry in children at risk of osteopenia. J Clin Densitom 2003;6:7–15.

51 Baroncelli GI, Federico G, Bertelloni S, Sodini F, de Terlizzi F, Cadossi R, Saggese G: Assessment of bone quality by quantitative ultrasound of proximal phalanges of the hand and fracture rate in children and adolescents with bone and mineral disorders. Pediatr Res 2003;54:125–136.

52 Larson CM, Henderson RC: Bone mineral density and fractures in boys with Duchenne muscular dystrophy. J Pediatr Orthop 2000;20:71–74.

53 Bachrach LK: Taking steps towards reducing osteoporosis in Duchenne muscular dystrophy. Neuromuscul Disord 2005;15:86–87.

54 Henderson RC, Specter BB: Kyphosis and fractures in children and young adults with cystic fibrosis. J Pediatr 1994;125:208–212.

55 Henderson RC, Lark RK, Gurka MJ, Worley G, Fung EB, Conaway M, Stallings VA, Stevenson RD: Bone density and metabolism in children and adolescents with moderate to severe cerebral palsy. Pediatrics 2002;110:e5.

56 Buison AM, Kawchak DA, Schall JI, Ohene-Frempong K, Stallings VA, Leonard MB, Zemel BS: Bone area and bone mineral content deficits in children with sickle cell disease. Pediatrics 2005;116:943–949.

57 McDonald DGM, Kinali M, Gallagher AC, Mercuri E, Muntoni F, Roper H, Jardine P, Jones DH, Pike MG: Fracture prevalence in Duchenne muscular dystrophy. Dev Med Child Neurol 2002;44:695–698.

58 Rovner AJ, Zemel BS, Leonard MB, Schall JI, Stallings VA: Mild to moderate cystic fibrosis is not associated with increased fracture risk in children and adolescents. J Pediatr 2005;147:327–331.

59 Mattson RH, Gidal BE: Fractures, epilepsy and antiepileptic drugs. Epilepsy Behav 2004;5:S36–S40.

60 Sheth RD: Bone health in pediatric epilepsy. Epilepsy Behav 2003;5:S30–S35.

61 Goulding A, Taylor RW, Jones IE, McAuley KA, Manning PJ, Williams SM: Overweight and obese children have low bone mass and area for their weight. Int J Obes 2000;24:627–632.

62 Goulding A, Taylor RW, Jones IE, Manning PJ, Williams SM: Spinal overload – a concern for obese children and adolescents? Osteoporos Int 2002;13:835–840.

63 Petit MA, Beck TJ, Shults J, Zemel BS, Foster BJ, Leonard MB: Proximal femur bone geometry is appropriately adapted to lean mass in overweight children and adolescents. Bone 2005;36:568–576.

64 Baroncelli GI, Bertelloni S, Sodini F, Saggese G: Lumbar bone mineral density at final height and prevalence of fractures in treated children with GH deficiency. J Clin Endocrinol Metab 2002;87:3624–3631.

65 Helenius I, Remes V, Salminen JJ, Vaita H, Makitie O, Holmberg C, Palmu P, Tervahartiala P, Sarna S, Helenius M, Peltonen J, Jalanko H: Incidence and predictors of fractures in children after solid organ transplantation. A 5-year prospective, population-based study. J Bone Miner Res 2006;21:380–387.

66 Leonard MB, Feldman HI, Shults J, Zemel BS, Foster B, Stallings V: Long-term, high-dose glucocorticoids and bone mineral content in childhood glucocorticoid-sensitive nephrotic syndrome. N Engl J Med 2004;351:868–875.

67 Bazelmans C, Coppieters Y, Godin I, Parent F, Berghmans L, Dramaix M, Leveque A: Is obesity associated with injuries among young people? Eur J Epidemiol 2004;19:1037–1042.

68 Goulding A, Jones IE, Taylor RW, Piggot JM, Taylor D: Dynamic and static tests of balance and postural sway in boys: effects of previous wrist bone fractures and high adiposity. Gait Posture 2003;17:136–141.

69 Daniels MW, Wilson DM, Paguntalan HG, Hoffman AR, Bachrach LK: Bone mineral density in pediatric transplant recipients. Transplantation 2003;76:673–678.

70 van der Sluis IM, van den Heuvel-Eibrink MM, Hablen K, Krenning EP, Kesizer-Schrama SMPFD: Altered bone mineral density and body composition, and increased fracture risk in childhood acute lymphoblastic leukemia. J Pediatr 2002;141:204–210.

71 Van Staa TP, Cooper C, Leufkens HGM, Bishop NJ: Children and the risk of fractures caused by oral corticosteroids. J Bone Miner Res 2003;18:913–918.

72 Van Staa TP, Bishop NJ, Leufkens HGM, Cooper C: Are inhaled corticosteroids associated with an increased risk of fracture in children? Osteoporos Int 2004;15:785–791.

73 Barnes C, Wong P, Egan B, Speller T, Cameron F, Jones G, Ekert H, Monagle P: Reduced bone density among children with severe hemophilia. Pediatrics 2004;114:e177–e181.

74 Caraballo PJ, Heit JA, Atkinson EJ, Silverstein MD, O'Fallon WM, Castro MR, Melton LJ: Long-term use of oral anticoagulants and the risk of fracture. Arch Int Med 1999;159:1750–1756.

75 Konstantynowicz J, Bialokoz-Kalinowska I, Motkowski R, Abramowicz P, Piotrowska-Jastrzebska J, Sienkiewicz J, Seeman E: The characteristics of fractures in Polish adolescents aged 16–20 years. Osteoporos Int 2005;16:1397–1403.

76 DiMeglio LA, Peacock M: Two-year clinical trial of oral alendronate versus intravenous pamidronate in children with osteogenesis imperfecta. J Bone Miner Res 2006;21:132–140.

77 Black RE, Williams SM, Jones IE, Goulding A: Children who avoid drinking cow milk have low dietary calcium intakes and poor bone health. Am J Clin Nutr 2002;76:675–680.

78 Cooper C, Javaid K, Westlake S, Harvey N, Dennison E: Developmental origins of osteoporotic fracture: the role of maternal vitamin D insufficiency. J Nutr 2005;135:2728S–2734S.

79 Demarini S: Calcium and phosphorus nutrition in preterm infants. Acta Paediatr 2005;94:87–92.

80 Cooper C, Westlake S, Harvey N, Javaid K, Dennison E, Hanson M: Review: developmental origins of osteoporotic fracture. Osteoporos Int 2006;17:337–347.

81 Matkovic V, Goel PK, Badenhop-Stevens NE, Landoll JD, Bin L, Ilich JZ, Skugor M, Nagode LA, Mobley SL, Ha E-J, Hangartner TN, Clairmont A: Calcium supplementation and bone mineral density in females from childhood to young adulthood: a randomized controlled trial. Am J Clin Nutr 2005;81:175–188.

82 Soyka LA, Grinspoon S, Levitsky LL, Herzog DB, Klibanski A: The effects of anorexia nervosa on bone metabolism in female adolescents. J Clin Endocrinol Metab 1999;84:4489–4496.

83 Grinspoon S, Thomas E, Pitts S, Gross E, Mickley D, Miller D, Herzog D, Klibanski A: Prevalence and predictive factors for regional osteopenia in women with anorexia nervosa. Ann Int Med 2000;133:790–794.

84 Welt CK, Chan JL, Bullen J, Murphy R, Smith P, DePaoli AM, Karalis A, Mantzoros CS: Recombinant human leptin in women with hypothalamic amenorrhea. N Engl J Med 2004;351:987–997.

85 Vestergaard P, Emborg C, Stoving RK, Hagen C, Mosekilde L, Brixen K: Fractures in patients with anorexia nervosa, bulimia nervosa, and other eating disorders – a nationwide register study. Int J Eat Disord 2002;32:301–308.

86 Wyshak G: Teenaged girls, carbonated beverage consumption, and bone fractures. Arch Pediatr Adolesc Med 2000;154:610–613.

87 Ma D, Jones G: Soft drink and milk consumption, physical activity, bone mass, and upper limb fractures in children: a population-based case-control study. Calcif Tissue Int 2004;75:286–291.

88 McGartland C, Robson PJ, Murray L, Cran G, Savage K, Watkins D, Rooney M, Boreham C: Carbonated soft drink consumption and bone mineral density in adolescence: the Northern Ireland Young Hearts Project. J Bone Min Res 2003;18:1563–1569.

89 Whiting SJ, Healey A, Psiuk S, Mirwald RL, Kowalski K, Bailey DA: Relationship between carbonated and other low nutrient dense beverages and bone mineral content of adolescents. Nutr Res 2001;21:1107–1115.

90 Goulding A: Milk components and bone health. Aust J Dairy Technol 2003;58:73–78.

91 Henderson RC, Hayes PR: Bone mineralization in children and adolescents with a milk allergy. Bone Miner 1994;27:1–12.

92 Stallings VA, Oddleifson NW, Negrini BY, Zemel BS, Wellens R: Bone mineral content and dietary calcium intake in children prescribed a low-lactose diet. J Pediatr Gastroenterol Nutr 1994;18:440–445.

93 Infante D, Tormo R: Risk of inadequate bone mineralization in diseases involving long-term suppression of dairy products. J Pediatr Gastroenterol Nutr 2000;30:310–313.

94 Hidvegi E, Arato A, Cserhati E, Horvath T, Szabo A, Szabo A: Slight decrease in bone mineralization in cow milk-sensitive children. J Pediatr Gastroenterol Nutr 2003;36:44–49.

95   Jensen VB, Jorgensen IM, Rasmussen KB, Molgaard C, Prahl P: Bone mineral status in children with cow milk allergy. Pediatr Allergy Immunol 2004;15:562–565.
96   Rockell JEP, Williams SM, Taylor RW, Grant AM, Jones IE, Goulding A: Two-year changes in bone and body composition in young children with a history of prolonged milk avoidance. Osteoporos Int 2005;16:1016–1023.
97   Manias K, McCabe D, Bishop N: Fractures and recurrent fractures in children; varying effects of environmental factors as well as bone size and mass. Bone 2006;39:652–657.
98   Kalkwarf HJ, Khoury JC, Lanphear BP: Milk intake during childhood and adolescence, adult bone density, and osteoporotic fractures in US women. Am J Clin Nutr 2003;77:257–265.
99   Di Stefano M, Veneto G, Malservisi S, Cecchetti L, Minguzzi L, Strocchi A, Corazza GR: Lactose malabsorption and intolerance and peak bone mass. Gastroenterology 2002;122:1793–1799.
100 Jesudason D, Need AG: Effects of smoking on bone and mineral metabolism. Endocrinologist 2002;12:199–209.
101 Vestergaard P, Mosekilde L: Fracture risk associated with smoking: a meta-analysis. J Int Med 2003;254:572–583.
102 Jones IE, Williams SM, Goulding A: Associations of birth weight and length, childhood size, and smoking with bone fractures during growth: evidence from a birth cohort study. Am J Epidemiol 2004;159:343–350.
103 Hassan I, Dorani BJ: Sports related fractures in children in north east England. Emerg Med J 2001;18:167–171.
104 Burt CW, Overpeck MD: Emergency visits for sports-related injuries. Ann Emerg Med 2001;37:301–308.
105 Idzikowski JR, Janes PC, Abbott PJ: Upper extremity snowboarding injuries – ten-year results from the Colorado snowboard injury survey. Am J Sports Med 2000;28:825–832.
106 Brudvik C, Hove LM: Childhood fractures in Bergen, Norway: identifying high-risk groups and activities. J Pediatr Orthop 2003;23:629–634.
107 Schieber RA, Branche-Dorsey CM, Ryan GW, Rutherford GW, Stevens JA, O'Neil J: Risk factors for injuries from in-line skating and the effectiveness of safety gear. N Engl J Med 1996;335:1630–1635.
108 Machold W, Kwasny O, Eisenhardt P, Kolonja A, Bauer E, Lehr S, Mayr W, Fuchs M: Reduction of severe wrist injuries in snowboarding by an optimized wrist protection device: a prospective randomized trial. J Trauma 2002;52:517–520.
109 Loder RT, Warschausky S, Schwartz EM, Hensinger RN, Greenfield ML: The psychosocial characteristics of children with fractures. J Pediatr Orthop 1995;15:41–46.
110 Ma DQ, Morley R, Jones G: Risk-taking, coordination and upper limb fractures in children: a population-based case-control study. Osteoporos Int 2004;15:633–638.
111 Lee YS, Low SL, Lim LA, Loke KY: Cyclic pamidronate infusion improves bone mineralisation and reduces fracture incidence in osteogenesis imperfecta. Eur J Pediatr 2001;160:641–644.
112 Sakkers R, Kok D, Engelbert R, van Dongen A, Jansen M, Pruijs H, Verbout A, Schweitzer D, Uiterwaal C: Skeletal effects and functional outcome with olpadronate in children with osteogenesis imperfecta: a 2-year randomised placebo-controlled trial. Lancet 2004;363:1427–1431.
113 Batch JA, Couper JJ, Rodda C, Cowell CT, Zacharin M: Use of bisphosphonate therapy for osteoporosis in childhood and adolescence. J Paediatr Child Health 2003;39:88–92.

Prof. Ailsa Goulding
Department of Medical and Surgical Sciences
University of Otago
Great King Street, PO Box 913
Dunedin 9054 (New Zealand)
Tel. +64 3 474 0999, ext. 8516, Fax +64 3 474 7641
E-Mail ailsa.goulding@stonebow.otago.ac.nz

Daly R, Petit M (eds): Optimizing Bone Mass and Strength. The Role of Physical Activity and
Nutrition during Growth. Med Sport Sci. Basel, Karger, 2007, vol 51, pp 121–136

....

Does Exercise during Growth Prevent Fractures in Later Life?

Magnus K. Karlsson

Clinical and Molecular Osteoporosis Research Unit, Department of Clinical Sciences,
Lund University, Malmö University Hospital, Malmö, Sweden

Abstract

Regular weight-bearing exercise, especially during the pre- or early peripubertal years,
leads to substantial benefits in bone mass and skeletal structure, enhancing bone strength at
loaded sites. However, few fragility fractures occur in young adulthood, and only if the exercise-
induced skeletal benefits are retained into older age, a time when the incidence of fragility fractures rises exponentially, would these changes be of biological significance for fracture reduction.
The limited data available indicate that exercise benefits in areal bone mineral density are eroded
in the long term. In contrast, several studies suggest that exercise-induced *structural* changes may
be retained even following the cessation of exercise. These structural changes may be more
important to overall bone strength than bone mass or density alone. In addition, residual benefits
in nonskeletal factors, such as improved muscle strength, coordination and balance, may also
reduce fracture risk. However, it is uncertain what actually happens to the fracture risk of individuals who retire from exercise and reduce their level of activity to that of the average individual.
Recent retrospective observational and case-control studies suggest that there could be a reduced
fracture risk in former athletes. However, since these studies are cross-sectional, no inferences
could be drawn as regards causality. Selection bias at baseline would actually produce the same
results. Furthermore, the biological explanation for the reduced fracture incidence is not clear
although several explanations have been proposed, including: residual benefits to bone structural
properties, muscle strength, coordination and balance. Each of these traits could be maintained in
former athletes after their active career, and may help to reduce the number of fractures later in
life. Therefore, based on the current evidence, we recommend a physically active lifestyle during
growth as a possible preventive strategy against fragility fractures in old age.

Copyright © 2007 S. Karger AG, Basel

The Fragility Fracture Problem

The incidence of fragility fractures has been rising for decades, so that
today an estimated 50% of all women and 30% of all men suffer a fracture

related to osteoporosis during their lifetime [1]. While there is currently no cure for osteoporosis, antiresorptive and bone-forming drugs are one approach to reduce the incidence of fractures; in women there is evidence that these drugs reduce fracture risk by about 50% [2], while the effect in men has not been well evaluated [2]. Importantly however, the fracture-protective effect is only shown in individuals with osteoporosis [3], with or without fragility fractures [2]. While the relative risk of a fracture is greatest in individuals with osteoporosis, most fractures in absolute numbers occur in the larger population of individuals at modestly increased risk because of modestly reduced areal bone mineral density (aBMD) or osteopenia [3]. In this group, the effect of drug treatment is less clear. Furthermore, general screening for detection of low aBMD is not considered to be cost-effective, as a modest deficit in aBMD implies a low absolute risk for sustaining a fracture [4]. Pharmacological treatment in these groups would involve treating a large number of individuals to prevent just one fracture event, an approach that is not particularly feasible or cost-effective. Thus, it is critical to develop community-based prevention strategies that are safe, accessible to all individuals, inexpensive to implement, without side effects, and that are effective in individuals with osteopenia as well as osteoporosis.

Physical activity is widely regarded as one strategy that may prevent fractures in later life. As noted in other chapters, physical activity, especially during childhood and adolescence, leads to bone modelling and remodelling changes that can optimize bone mass, bone geometry, and ultimately the mechanical strength of bone. However, these benefits may be transient, that is, the exercise-induced benefits in aBMD during growth may be eroded by cessation of exercise [5, 6]. In contrast, exercise-induced changes in bone size and shape (periosteal expansion) may be permanent, [7–9] and thus may fulfil the criteria for a future fracture-preventive tool. However, it is uncertain whether physical activity during the growing years really creates beneficial skeletal changes that are retained into later life. Perhaps more importantly, does this strategy really reduce fracture risk in old age? If the skeletal benefits of exercise derived during childhood, adolescence or young adulthood are totally eroded by time, then should exercise during childhood be used as a prevention strategy for fracture reduction? Having a high aBMD during the growing years does not influence fracture frequency during this period as healthy children usually do not suffer a fracture related to osteoporosis even if they have a low aBMD. If the aim is to reduce the fracture burden in the community, then physical activity must confer long-term benefits on the skeleton into older age.

Exercise could also lead to nonskeletal benefits such as a higher muscle mass, and improved coordination and balance, benefits that hypothetically could reduce the fracture incidence even if no residual skeletal benefits are retained. Thus, we must aim to evaluate the effect of exercise by using the clinically relevant end point, fracture, not only aBMD or bone structure. The purpose of this chapter is to examine the hypothesis that exercise during childhood, adolescence and young adulthood leads to increased bone strength, even in a long-term perspective, and reduces the risk of fragility fracture in old age. Specifically, we address the following questions: (1) does exercise during growth increase the accrual of bone mass and improve bone structure? (2) are exercise-induced benefits to aBMD and bone structure retained following the cessation of training? and (3) what is the role of childhood and adolescent activity on fragility fractures in later life? Throughout this chapter, differences presented are significant unless otherwise stated.

Does Exercise during Growth Increase the Accrual of Bone Mass and Improve Bone Structure?

As discussed in other chapters, exercise during growth is more osteogenic than the same physical activity undertaken during adulthood [10–16]. This view is supported by the results from both animal and human studies. For instance, the mechanical threshold for bone to respond to loading in old rats was found to be higher than in young rats but, once activated, the cells of the older rats had the same capacity to respond to loading as the younger rats [17]. However, the relative bone formation rate and the relative bone-forming surface were less in old compared to young rats under similar loads [17, 18]. These data are supported by evidence that the responsiveness of mature bone is less in old compared to young turkeys exposed to a similar load [19].

Human studies also support the view that immature bone is more responsive to loading than mature bone. Cross-sectional studies in young tennis players report that the side-to-side differences in bone mass are up to four times higher in female players who began training 5 years before menarche than in those starting 15 years after menarche [20]. Prospective and retrospective cohort studies also indicate that physically active children have higher aBMD than sedentary controls [21]. For example, prepubertal gymnasts involved in regular high-impact weight-bearing activities have 10–30% higher aBMD than controls, with the greatest difference reported in the arms, a weight-bearing site in these athletes [22]. These differences in favor of exercising or athletic children are much larger in magnitude than the difference achieved by exercise during adulthood. Although many of these studies are often confounded by selection bias, the results from a limited number of prospective controlled trials support the notion that exercise during growth may help to build a stronger skeleton that is more resistant to trauma. To date, there have been eight controlled intervention studies of varying duration (some randomized and some nonrandomized) that have been performed on pre-, peri- and postpubertal boys and girls [10, 12–14] (discussed in detail in the chapters by Daly, this vol., pp. 33–49 and Hughes et al., this vol., pp. 137–158). These studies have reported that a moderate weight-bearing exercise intervention in the prepubertal and early pubertal years confers significant skeletal benefits [10, 12–15, 16], whereas a similar training program conducted in postpubertal children does not appear to enhance bone mineral accrual [23–25]. One of these intervention studies followed children for 4 years with daily moderate exercise in the intervention group [16, 26]. In this study, exercise enhanced both bone mass and structure, which highlights that regular weight-bearing exercise during growth can lead to long-term benefits in terms of skeletal health [27]. In summary, these data imply that physical activity, even at a moderate level that is possible for all children to participate in, confers skeletal benefits for both the accrual of bone mineral and the skeletal structure.

Are Exercise-Induced Benefits to Areal Bone Mineral Density Retained following the Cessation of Training?

Animal studies generally indicate that benefits to bone mass and structure are lost with cessation of the training program. One randomized controlled prospective trial involving 50 young rats allocated to 8 or 12 weeks of training followed by 4 weeks of detraining revealed that femoral wet weight, bone volume, cross-sectional area and cortical area all increased with the training regime, but that all benefits were lost with the 4 weeks of detraining [28]. Another trial in rats reported that there were residual short-term benefits in aBMD following training [29], but again all benefits were lost following a longer period of detraining [30]. In contrast, a recent study in young rats showed that exercise during early adolescence enhanced bone structure and that these benefits were maintained throughout life [31].

Are Exercise-Induced Benefits in Bone Mass Preserved with Retirement?

How are skeletal changes reflected in humans who have retired from sports? Studies using biochemical markers of bone turnover suggest that reduced activity leads to increased rates of bone resorption, supporting the idea that benefits may be lost (or at least reduced) with cessation of activity. When comparing active soccer players with retired players [32], just 2 weeks of detraining was found to be associated with an increase in bone resorption markers and a decrease in bone formation markers [33]. At present, we only have short-term prospective data that have monitored changes in bone mass, density and structure with retirement from physical activity. There are also few published long-term cross-sectional studies, all of which are subject to the risk of selection bias. Most of these studies are retrospective analyses using aBMD as a surrogate end point. It is also important to recognize that a cross-sectional study design can draw no inferences with regard to causality. Stronger individuals, those with a large muscle mass and an accompanying higher aBMD, may choose to do more sport during childhood and adolescence, while less athletic individuals may choose to be less active because of their reduced physical ability and their lack of success in sports, a phenotype that is typically characterized by a low bone mass or density. Thus, the causal link could be between the phenotype with high aBMD, larger muscle mass and strength, success in sports and the low incidence of fragility fracture, rather than a direct effect of the exercise itself on risk of fragility fractures.

Published data both support and oppose the possibility that exercise is associated with benefits in aBMD that are maintained after cessation of exercise [5–7, 34–42]. One cross-sectional trial in tennis players showed that the side-to-side difference in bone mineral content remained in athletes who had reduced their training, suggesting that the benefits in bone mineral content were maintained with reduced activity level [7]. However, these data should be interpreted cautiously due to the small sample size, the high recreational activity level at follow-up and the short detraining period. The prospective reports that support the maintenance of aBMD benefits following the cessation of exercise also have limitations with respect to the study design. Some studies do not include more than 12 retired athletes; others include retired athletes still involved in a higher than average activity level; all studies have followed the former athletes for only a short period into retirement, and in one study there were actually some skeletal regions with a higher aBMD loss in athletes than in controls [34, 39–42]. As such, these results must be regarded as promising but not conclusive, and before we can draw more definite conclusions, these cohorts should be followed for a longer period of retirement.

When examining the available prospective data from a longer perspective of retirement, our inferences are less promising. In one of the first prospective reports which included 23 middle-aged male and female runners aged 55–77 years at baseline, Michel et al. [43] reported that after 5 years the loss in spine aBMD was 13% in those who stopped running in comparison to 4% in those who continued to run. Similar results were reported in a short-term intervention evaluating the influence of unilateral leg press four times per week for 12 months in 12 women aged 19–27 years. Following the 12-month training period, there was a 2% nonsignificant increase in aBMD, but 3 months of detraining was followed by a return of aBMD to the pretraining levels [44]. However, since this study only included 12 women, it is difficult to draw any definitive conclusions. In a similar study involving 29 premenopausal women who completed a 12-month exercise training program, significant increases were observed in aBMD relative to 22 controls at the completion of the intervention, but all these benefits were lost with 12 months of detraining [45]. There are now also two larger prospective controlled studies that have followed former athletes for 5–8 years into retirement [5, 6]: the first including 97 male ice hockey and soccer players and 49 controls [5], and the second including 66 female soccer players and 64 controls [6]. Both studies reported that the athletes at baseline had a 1.0–1.5 SD higher aBMD than controls. However, after 4–5 years of retirement, the remaining exercise-induced benefits in aBMD were reduced by half. These two studies also revealed that the loss in aBMD following retirement was greater than the changes in both the athletes who proceeded with exercise and in the controls. In spite of these higher rates of bone loss, aBMD remained higher in the retired athletes than in the controls but at a lower level than during their active career.

When evaluating the effect of retirement on bone health over many decades, including the ages where the incidence of fragility fracture rises exponentially, we must rely on cross-sectional data. One trial of 22 active and 128 formerly active male soccer players and 138 controls showed that the former athletes had higher aBMD than controls during the first two decades after retirement. However, the magnitude of the difference in aBMD was lower in retired athletes than in active soccer players [46]. The estimated diminution in leg aBMD from these cross-sectional data was 0.33% per year in the former soccer players, around 50% higher that the 0.21% diminution per year in controls (fig. 1). Athletes who had been retired for 5 years still had a 10% higher leg aBMD than age-matched controls; those retired for 16 years still had a 5% higher leg aBMD, but there was no apparent aBMD benefit for players retired for 42 years (fig. 1) [46]. No benefits were seen at the hip, spine or any other skeletal region. Cross-sectional data in former female soccer players support these findings. Twenty-five former female soccer players aged 40 years and retired for 10 years were found to have higher aBMD, although less than during their active career [47]. Unfortunately, these female athletes were not followed over a longer period, so whether any residual benefits were sustained after age 65 could not be determined. In former male weight lifters, total body aBMD was found to be higher after retirement from an active career; 8% when they were 35–49 years old; 6% when they were 50–64 years old, but no higher when they were 65–79 years compared to controls [35–37]. Similar data are also reported in retired professional male and female ballet dancers both in Australia [48] and in Sweden (fig. 2) [38] as well as in retired Australian gymnasts [22].

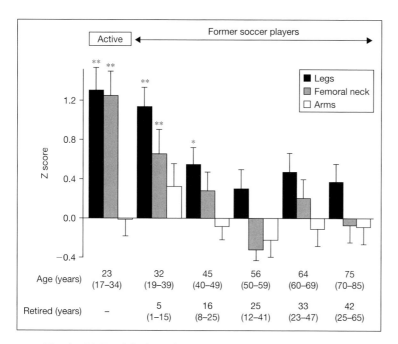

Fig. 1. aBMD of the legs, femoral neck and arms in active and formerly active male soccer players and controls in relation to age. aBMD in the active and former athletes is presented as Z scores (number of SD difference compared to age- and gender-matched controls) in groups with advancing age and increased time since retirement from active exercise career. Bars represent means $\pm$ SD. *p $<$ 0.05; **p $<$ 0.01.

In summary, most of the available data regarding the long-term residual effects of exercise on bone health are based on cross-sectional studies, which makes interpretation difficult. Most longitudinal studies report a higher loss in aBMD in former athletes than in controls and cross-sectional data including old former athletes also indicate a higher loss in aBMD with aging (and time since retirement) than in controls. There is also evidence that aBMD in old former athletes is no different from controls, and thus it would seem that there are no long-term residual benefits found in aBMD in old and elderly former athletes. However, it must be recognized that there are studies that support the view that exercise-induced benefits during growth can, at least partly, be retained with a lower level of exercise [46], but secular trends in these cross-sectional studies are also important to consider when interpreting these results. Training during growth several decades ago may have been less vigorous, so it is possible that the now older retired athletes did not have the same magnitude of skeletal benefit as active athletes today. A different lifestyle after cessation of exercise

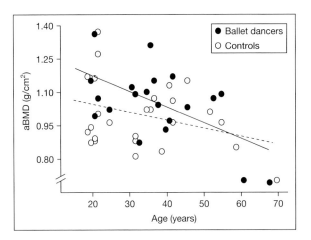

Fig. 2. aBMD of the femoral neck in active and former active female ballet dancers and in controls in relation to age. The slopes differ significantly (p < 0.05) when the groups are compared. Adapted from Karlsson et al. [38].

compared to controls may also influence outcomes. More sedentary living in retirement, lower workloads and less recreational physical activity or greater intake of alcohol are all factors that could affect aBMD in adult life. That said, most of the published studies have reported virtually no differences in workload, lifestyle, recreational activity, smoking habits, alcohol consumption and nutritional habits between former athletes and controls as assessed by questionnaires [35–38, 46]. Nonetheless, these are important factors to consider when interpreting these data. Clearly further prospective studies are needed to fully address these important questions.

Are Exercise-Induced Structural Changes of the Skeleton Preserved with Retirement?

Most of the studies cited in the previous section have only evaluated changes in aBMD following retirement from sports. Even if all the benefits in aBMD are lost with detraining, there is a possibility that any structural changes induced by exercise during growth could be retained. The enlargement in bone size in the playing arm of former tennis players was maintained with cessation of exercise, despite a lack of difference in volumetric BMD [7]. Twelve former adult male tennis players who had been retired for 1–3 years had higher humeral shaft side-to-side differences in peripheral quantitative computed tomography-derived total cross-sectional area (13%), cortical area (23%), bone strength index (24%), principal moments of inertia (41%) and cortical wall thickness (20%) compared to controls [7]. The marrow cavity was also larger in the playing arm of the former players, suggesting that there was either greater endocortical expansion during activity or a higher endocortical resorption after retirement. These observations are consistent with the hypothesis that exercise produces enlargement of bone size that is permanent, but that the increased bone mass through endocortical apposition may be lost with retirement. The same view was supported in a randomized controlled prospective trial involving 239 children aged 3–5 years [9]. Twelve months of physical activity resulted in both periosteal and endosteal expansion, and these benefits relative to controls remained following 12 months of detraining. These structural changes are likely to be of significant biological importance, as placing the cortical shell further away from the center of a tubular bone increases bone strength by the fourth power of the radius [49]. In a cross-sectional study of 90 former male soccer players and weight lifters aged 50–92 who had been retired for 3–65 years, bone size at the femoral neck and lumbar spine was greater than in 77 sedentary age- and gender-matched controls [8]. However, the estimate of bone size in this study was derived from dual-energy X-ray absorptiometry (DXA), a two-dimensional imaging technique which could misinterpret the actual bone size. Despite these concerns, there were also remaining benefits in quantitative ultrasound parameters in the old former athletes; quantitative ultrasound is reported to estimate not only the quantity of bone mineral, but also the quality or the skeletal architecture [50], a trait not captured by DXA. These latter data indicate that exercise-induced structural skeletal changes, not captured in aBMD assessed by DXA, may be preserved in former athletes into old age. If so, changes in bone dimensions or structure could help reduce the risk of fragility fracture. However, before we can draw conclusive inferences, these traits must be assessed both in prospectively followed cohorts and in long-term evaluated cross-sectional trials.

Influence of Current Physical Activity and Detraining on Fracture Risk

There are no prospective controlled studies that evaluate the role of child-hood or adolescent physical activity on fragility fractures in later life. Due to the complexity and expense of performing such a trial, it is unlikely these trials will be done. Most fractures occur as a result of a fall. However, the low absolute incidence of falls with an even lower incidence of fractures among the fallers makes it extremely difficult to create randomized exercise intervention studies with fractures as the end point. When designing a study with hip fracture as the end point, a 5-year study with an α level equal to 0.05 and a β coefficient equal to 0.20; a control group with a hip fracture incidence among 75-year-old women of 3–6% over a 5-year period and with risk reduction of 25% with exercise, and sample sizes close to 7,000 individuals are needed to achieve the statistical power to detect a fracture-reducing effect of exercise. Moreover, due to the expected large proportions of dropouts and nonresponders, a further 25% increase in the groups could be recommended [51]. This is the reason why we have to rely on studies with a lower level of evidence within the evidence-based hierarchy when drawing inferences with regard to exercise and fracture risk. It must also be emphasized that retrospective and prospective observational and case-control studies consistently suggest that a high current level of physical activity is associated with a low hip fracture risk in both men and women [51, 52]. Finding a dose-response relationship between the current activity level and the risk reduction further strengthens this view [53]. However, there are little data evaluating the importance of the current activity level on the incidence of nonhip fractures or more specifically low-energy fractures related to osteoporosis. The few studies that have addressed this question have reported both a significant and nonsignificant lower fracture risk in individuals with a high current level of physical activity compared to those with lower levels of activity [51, 52].

The final and perhaps most important question is what happens to the risk of fracture after a period of high-level physical training is followed by lower levels of physical activity. There are few published studies, all cross-sectional, that have addressed this question. One study of 284 retired male soccer players (48 years and over) and age- and gender-matched controls (n = 568) showed no difference in the incidence of any fracture (all types of fractures included; 20 vs. 21%) or in fragility fracture incidence (2 vs. 4%) between controls and soccer players [46]. However, in absolute values, the proportion of individuals with a fragility fracture in the former soccer players was half that of the controls, but the sample size in this study was relatively small and thus there is an increased likelihood of a type II error. As a result, the study sample was extended, and an increase in the study population led the researchers to change their conclusions. With the inclusion of 663 former elite athletes aged 50–94 years who were involved in impact-loading sport and had been retired for 1–62 years, and 943 gender- and age-matched controls, there was no difference in the proportion of individuals with regard to the lifetime risk of fractures (26 vs. 25% of the individuals) (fig. 3) [5]. In contrast, after retirement from sports, there were significantly fewer former athletes with fractures than controls (8.9 vs. 12.1%). There were also significantly fewer former athletes with fragility fractures sustained after age 50 years (2.3 vs. 4.2%), and fewer former athletes with distal radius fractures (0.8 vs. 2.3%) (fig. 3) [5]. In 400 former male soccer

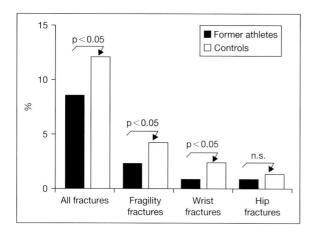

Fig. 3. Proportion of individuals with fractures among 663 former male athletes now aged 50–94 years and in 943 age- and gender-matched controls. The figure includes the lifetime risk of sustaining a fracture, the risk of sustaining a fracture after age 35 (after retirement) and the risk of sustaining a fragility fracture, a wrist fracture and a hip fracture after age 50 due to a low-energy trauma. Adapted from Nordstrom et al. [5].

players now aged 60–94 years and 800 controls, similar results were found with virtually the same proportions of individuals with fractures [8]. Together, these findings confirm that there is an association between physical activity early in life and fracture risk in old age (fig. 4). However, in spite of these promising data, it is important to recognize that these studies can draw no conclusions as regards causality. Residual nonskeletal benefits in the former athletes, such as neuromuscular function, coordination, balance and fall frequency, as well as selection bias and differences in lifestyle habits during adulthood relative to the controls may all explain the outcome.

There is also one study which has reported that exercise during growth is not associated with a low fracture risk in old age. In a large observational study, Wyshak et al. [54] reported a greater lifetime risk of sustaining any fractures in 2,622 former female college athletes aged 20–80 years compared to 2,776 age- and gender-matched controls (41 vs. 32%), but the number of individuals with fractures were similar between retired athletes and controls (29 vs. 32%). However, it is difficult to draw any definitive conclusions from this study because the sample included women from age 20 years, some with an extremely short period of retirement, and many who were currently involved in a range of different physical activities, including both impact- and non-impact-loaded sports.

Currently, there are no studies that fulfil the demands of a randomized prospective exercise intervention trial evaluating the effect of retirement with

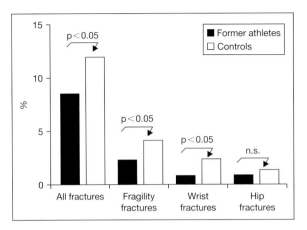

Fig. 4. Proportion of individuals with fractures among 400 former male soccer players now aged 60–94 years and in 800 age- and gender-matched controls. The figure includes the lifetime risk of sustaining a fracture, the risk of sustaining a fracture after age 35 (after retirement) and the risk of sustaining a fragility fracture, a wrist fracture and a hip fracture after age 50 due to a low-energy trauma. Adapted from Karlsson et al. [8].

fractures as the end point. There is, however, one study with a similar study design [55]. Twenty-seven postmenopausal women aged 58–75 were subjected to a 2-year back-strengthening program and compared with 23 controls. The intervention resulted in improved back strength in the exercising women but not a higher aBMD. All women were then reevaluated 8 years after the intervention. The women in the intervention group still had a higher back muscle strength, but also a higher aBMD and fewer spine fractures [14 fractures in 322 vertebral bodies examined (4.3%) in the control group and 6 fractures in 378 vertebral bodies examined (1.6%) in the intervention group]. The relative risk of compression fracture was 2.7 times greater in the control group than in the intervention group. To our knowledge, this is the first and only study reported in the literature demonstrating a possible long-term effect of strengthening the back muscles on the reduction of vertebral fractures [55]. However, this study did not evaluate clinically relevant vertebral fractures, only radiographically defined vertebral deformities, and the statistical calculation was based on the number of vertebral bodies evaluated and the number of vertebrae with a fracture, not the number of individuals with a fracture. As a result, it is difficult to draw conclusions with prudence, and trials with a similar study design using the number of individuals with fractures and clinical fractures as end point (that is, fractures leading to back pain) must first be published before we can finally answer the research question with stronger evidence.

Summary and Conclusion

The current published data suggest that physical activity during growth is associated with a beneficial effect on aBMD and bone structure. However, data from both cross-sectional studies of old former athletes and a limited number of longitudinal studies indicate that cessation of exercise appears to be associated with a greater rate of bone loss (at least from aBMD outcomes), and thus it seems that in the long term any initial benefits to aBMD will be lost in later life. In contrast, exercise-induced benefits in skeletal size, shape and structure may be permanent. These changes in bone size and shape are more important to the overall strength of the skeleton than the measurable changes in aBMD. The finding that fewer former athletes sustain all types of fractures and fragility fractures after retirement from participation in high-level physical activity provides some evidence that exercise during the first two decades of life could have long-term beneficial effects on the skeleton or factors related to falls into old age. Until further rigorous research is conducted, we must rely on the present evidence and continue to recommend physical activity during growth as a possible means to help prevent fractures in old age.

References

1   Cooper C, Campion G, Melton LJ 3rd: Hip fractures in the elderly: a world-wide projection. Osteoporos Int 1992;2:285–289.
2   Karlsson MK, Gerdhem P, Ahlborg HG: The prevention of osteoporotic fractures. J Bone Joint Surg Br 2005;87:1320–1327.
3   World Health Organization: Assessment of fracture risk and its application to screening for postmenopausal osteoporosis. Report of a WHO Study Group. World Health Organ Tech Rep Ser 1994;843:1–129.
4   SBU95. The Swedish Council on Technology Assessment in Health Care: Measurement of Bone Density. SBU Report No 127. Stockholm, 1995.
5   Nordstrom A, Karlsson C, Nyquist F, Olsson T, Nordstrom P, Karlsson M: Bone loss and fracture risk after reduced physical activity. J Bone Miner Res 2005;20:202–207.
6   Valdimarsson O, Ahlborg HG, Duppe H, Nyquist F, Karlsson M: Reduced training is associated with increased loss of BMD. J Bone Miner Res 2005;20:906–912.
7   Haapasalo H, Kontulainen S, Sievanen H, Kannus P, Jarvinen M, Vuori I: Exercise-induced bone gain is due to enlargement in bone size without a change in volumetric bone density: a peripheral quantitative computed tomography study of the upper arms of male tennis players. Bone 2000;27: 351–357.
8   Karlsson MK, Alborg HG, Obrant K, Nyquist F, Lindberg H, Karlsson C: Exercise during growth and young adulthood is associated with reduced fracture risk in old ages. J Bone Miner Res 2002;17(suppl 1):S297.
9   Specker B, Binkley T, Fahrenwald N: Increased periosteal circumference remains present 12 months after an exercise intervention in preschool children. Bone 2004;35:1383–1388.
10 Bradney M, Pearce G, Naughton G, Sullivan C, Bass S, Beck T, Carlson J, Seeman E: Moderate exercise during growth in prepubertal boys: changes in bone mass, size, volumetric density, and bone strength: a controlled prospective study. J Bone Miner Res 1998;13:1814–1821.

11   Karlsson M, Bass S, Seeman E: The evidence that exercise during growth or adulthood reduces the risk of fragility fractures is weak. Best Pract Res Clin Rheumatol 2001;15:429–450.

12   MacKelvie KJ, Khan KM, Petit MA, Janssen PA, McKay HA: A school-based exercise intervention elicits substantial bone health benefits: a 2-year randomized controlled trial in girls. Pediatrics 2003;112:e447.

13   MacKelvie KJ, McKay HA, Khan KM, Crocker PR: A school-based exercise intervention augments bone mineral accrual in early pubertal girls. J Pediatr 2001;139:501–508.

14   MacKelvie KJ, McKay HA, Petit MA, Moran O, Khan KM: Bone mineral response to a 7-month randomized controlled, school-based jumping intervention in 121 prepubertal boys: associations with ethnicity and body mass index. J Bone Miner Res 2002;17:834–844.

15   McKay HA, Petit MA, Schutz RW, Prior JC, Barr SI, Khan KM: Augmented trochanteric bone mineral density after modified physical education classes: a randomized school-based exercise intervention study in prepubescent and early pubescent children. J Pediatr 2000;136:156–162.

16   Valdimarsson O, Linden C, Johnell O, Gardsell P, Karlsson MK: Daily physical education in the school curriculum in prepubertal girls during 1 year is followed by an increase in bone mineral accrual and bone width – data from the prospective controlled Malmo pediatric osteoporosis prevention study. Calcif Tissue Int 2006;78:65–71.

17   Turner CH, Takano Y, Owan I: Aging changes mechanical loading thresholds for bone formation in rats. J Bone Miner Res 1995;10:1544–1549.

18   Turner CH, Forwood MR, Rho JY, Yoshikawa T: Mechanical loading thresholds for lamellar and woven bone formation. J Bone Miner Res 1994;9:87–97.

19   Rubin CT, Bain SD, McLeod KJ: Suppression of the osteogenic response in the aging skeleton. Calcif Tissue Int 1992;50:306–313.

20   Kannus P, Haapasalo H, Sankelo M, Sievanen H, Pasanen M, Heinonen A, Oja P, Vuori I: Effect of starting age of physical activity on bone mass in the dominant arm of tennis and squash players. Ann Intern Med 1995;123:27–31.

21   Bailey DA, McKay HA, Mirwald RL, Crocker PR, Faulkner RA: A six-year longitudinal study of the relationship of physical activity to bone mineral accrual in growing children: the University of Saskatchewan bone mineral accrual study. J Bone Miner Res 1999;14:1672–1679.

22   Bass S, Pearce G, Bradney M, Hendrich E, Delmas PD, Harding A, Seeman E: Exercise before puberty may confer residual benefits in bone density in adulthood: studies in active prepubertal and retired female gymnasts. J Bone Miner Res 1998;13:500–507.

23   Fuchs RK, Bauer JJ, Snow CM: Jumping improves hip and lumbar spine bone mass in prepubescent children: a randomized controlled trial. J Bone Miner Res 2001;16:148–156.

24   Heinonen A, Sievanen H, Kannus P, Oja P, Pasanen M, Vuori I: High-impact exercise and bones of growing girls: a 9-month controlled trial. Osteoporos Int 2000;11:1010–1017.

25   Morris FL, Naughton GA, Gibbs JL, Carlson JS, Wark JD: Prospective ten-month exercise intervention in premenarcheal girls: positive effects on bone and lean mass. J Bone Miner Res 1997;12:1453–1462.

26   Linden C, Gardsell P, Ahlborg HG, Karlsson MK: A school curriculum-based exercise program increases bone mineral accrual in boys and girls during early adolescence – four-year data from the POP study (pediatric preventive osteoporotic study). J Bone Miner Res 2005;20:S4.

27   Lindén C, Stenevi-Lundgren S, Gardsell P, Karlsson MK: A five-year school curriculum-based exercise program in girls during early adolescence is associated with a large bone size and a thick cortical shell – pQCT data from the Prospective Pediatric Osteoporosis Prevention Study (POP study). J Bone Miner Res 2006;21:S38.

28   Iwamoto J, Yeh JK, Aloia JF: Effect of deconditioning on cortical and cancellous bone growth in the exercise trained young rats. J Bone Miner Res 2000;15:1842–1849.

29   Jarvinen TL, Pajamaki I, Sievanen H, Vuohelainen T, Tuukkanen J, Jarvinen M, Kannus P: Femoral neck response to exercise and subsequent deconditioning in young and adult rats. J Bone Miner Res 2003;18:1292–1299.

30   Pajamaki I, Kannus P, Vuohelainen T, Sievanen H, Tuukkanen J, Jarvinen M, Jarvinen TL: The bone gain induced by exercise in puberty is not preserved through a virtually life-long deconditioning: a randomized controlled experimental study in male rats. J Bone Miner Res 2003;18: 544–552.

31   Warden SJ, Fuchs RK, Castillo AB, Turner CH: Does exercise during growth influence osteoporotic fracture risk later in life? J Musculoskelet Neuronal Interact 2005;5:344–346.

32 Karlsson KM, Karlsson C, Ahlborg HG, Valdimarsson O, Ljunghall S: The duration of exercise as a regulator of bone turnover. Calcif Tissue Int 2003;73:350–355.

33 Karlsson KM, Karlsson C, Ahlborg HG, Valdimarsson O, Ljunghall S, Obrant KJ: Bone turnover responses to changed physical activity. Calcif Tissue Int 2003;72:675–680.

34 Heinonen A, Kannus P, Sievanen H, Pasanen M, Oja P, Vuori I: Good maintenance of high-impact activity-induced bone gain by voluntary, unsupervised exercises: an 8-month follow-up of a randomized controlled trial. J Bone Miner Res 1999;14:125–128.

35 Karlsson MK, Hasserius R, Obrant KJ: Bone mineral density in athletes during and after career: a comparison between loaded and unloaded skeletal regions. Calcif Tissue Int 1996;59:245–248.

36 Karlsson MK, Johnell O, Obrant KJ: Is bone mineral density advantage maintained long-term in previous weight lifters? Calcif Tissue Int 1995;57:325–328.

37 Karlsson MK, Johnell O, Obrant KJ: Bone mineral density in weight lifters. Calcif Tissue Int 1993;52:212–215.

38 Karlsson MK, Johnell O, Obrant KJ: Bone mineral density in professional ballet dancers. Bone Miner 1993;21:163–169.

39 Kontulainen S, Kannus P, Haapasalo H, Heinonen A, Sievanen H, Oja P, Vuori I: Changes in bone mineral content with decreased training in competitive young adult tennis players and controls: a prospective 4-year follow-up. Med Sci Sports Exerc 1999;31:646–652.

40 Kontulainen S, Kannus P, Haapasalo H, Sievanen H, Pasanen M, Heinonen A, Oja P, Vuori I: Good maintenance of exercise-induced bone gain with decreased training of female tennis and squash players: a prospective 5-year follow-up study of young and old starters and controls. J Bone Miner Res 2001;16:195–201.

41 Kontulainen SA, Kannus PA, Pasanen ME, Sievanen HT, Heinonen AO, Oja P, Vuori I: Does previous participation in high-impact training result in residual bone gain in growing girls? One-year follow-up of a 9-month jumping intervention. Int J Sports Med 2002;23:575–581.

42 Kontulainen S, Heinonen A, Kannus P, Pasanen M, Sievanen H, Vuori I: Former exercisers of an 18-month intervention display residual aBMD benefits compared with control women 3.5 years post-intervention: a follow-up of a randomized controlled high-impact trial. Osteoporos Int 2004;15:248–251.

43 Michel BA, Lane NE, Bjorkengren A, Bloch DA, Fries JF: Impact of running on lumbar bone density: a 5-year longitudinal study. J Rheumatol 1992;19:1759–1763.

44 Vuori I, Heinonen A, Sievanen H, Kannus P, Pasanen M, Oja P: Effects of unilateral strength training and detraining on bone mineral density and content in young women: a study of mechanical loading and deloading on human bones. Calcif Tissue Int 1994;55:59–67.

45 Winters KM, Snow CM: Detraining reverses positive effects of exercise on the musculoskeletal system in premenopausal women. J Bone Miner Res 2000;15:2495–2503.

46 Karlsson MK, Linden C, Karlsson C, Johnell O, Obrant K, Seeman E: Exercise during growth and bone mineral density and fractures in old age. Lancet 2000;355:469–470.

47 Duppe H, Gardsell P, Johnell O, Ornstein E: Bone mineral density in female junior, senior and former football players. Osteoporos Int 1996;6:437–441.

48 Khan KM, Green RM, Saul A, Bennell KL, Crichton KJ, Hopper JL, Wark JD: Retired elite female ballet dancers and nonathletic controls have similar bone mineral density at weightbearing sites. J Bone Miner Res 1996;11:1566–1574.

49 Ahlborg HG, Johnell O, Turner CH, Rannevik G, Karlsson MK: Bone loss and bone size after menopause. N Engl J Med 2003;349:327–334.

50 Karlsson MK, Duan Y, Ahlborg H, Obrant KJ, Johnell O, Seeman E: Age, gender, and fragility fractures are associated with differences in quantitative ultrasound independent of bone mineral density. Bone 2001;28:118–122.

51 Gregg EW, Cauley JA, Seeley DG, Ensrud KE, Bauer DC: Physical activity and osteoporotic fracture risk in older women. Study of Osteoporotic Fractures Research Group. Ann Intern Med 1998;129:81–88.

52 Gregg EW, Pereira MA, Caspersen CJ: Physical activity, falls, and fractures among older adults: a review of the epidemiologic evidence. J Am Geriatr Soc 2000;48:883–893.

53   Coupland C, Wood D, Cooper C: Physical inactivity is an independent risk factor for hip fracture in the elderly. J Epidemiol Community Health 1993;47:441–443.
54   Wyshak G, Frisch RE, Albright TE, Albright NL, Schiff I: Bone fractures among former college athletes compared with nonathletes in the menopausal and postmenopausal years. Obstet Gynecol 1987;69:121–126.
55   Sinaki M, Itoi E, Wahner HW, Wollan P, Gelzcer R, Mullan BP, Collins DA, Hodgson SF: Stronger back muscles reduce the incidence of vertebral fractures: a prospective 10-year follow-up of post-menopausal women. Bone 2002;30:836–841.

Prof. Magnus Karlsson, MD, PhD
Clinical and Molecular Osteoporosis Research Unit
Department of Clinical Sciences
Lund University
Malmö University Hospital
SE–205 02 Malmö (Sweden)
Tel. +46 40 331000, Fax +46 40 336200
E-Mail magnus.karlsson@med.lu.se

Daly R, Petit M (eds): Optimizing Bone Mass and Strength. The Role of Physical Activity and Nutrition during Growth. Med Sport Sci. Basel, Karger, 2007, vol 51, pp 137–158

....

Lessons Learned from School-Based Skeletal Loading Intervention Trials: Putting Research into Practice

Julie M. Hughes, Susan A. Novotny, Rachel J. Wetzsteon, Moira A. Petit

School of Kinesiology, University of Minnesota, Minneapolis, Minn., USA

Abstract

In recent years, there have been a number of school-based physical activity intervention trials aimed at optimizing bone development. Various approaches have been taken including interventions ranging from 3 to 50 min in length performed 2–5 times per week incorporated within the school day (typically in physical education) or as an after-school program. Overall, these studies showed that school-based skeletal loading interventions are efficacious, safe, and feasible. Furthermore, studies to date have shown that interventions are most effective when initiated during prepuberty and early puberty, and consist of dynamic activities that are high in magnitude (i.e. jumping, skipping, hopping) and include multidirectional movements. Recent work also suggests that adding rest intervals and performing short bouts of activity a few times per day may enhance the effectiveness of loading on bone health. In this chapter, we discuss important training principles and lessons learned from these intervention trials and provide practical guidelines, tips and sample programs that can be used by health care professionals interested in optimizing bone health of children and adolescents.

Copyright © 2007 S. Karger AG, Basel

An estimated 200 million people worldwide have osteoporosis, and the prevalence is predicted to increase at an epidemic rate with the aging population. To counteract this alarming trend, it is important to identify interventions that can be implemented at the population level to optimize bone health. In order to be successful, population level interventions should be efficacious, widely available, time effective, economical, safe and enjoyable. Physical activity has the potential to meet these criteria.

As reviewed in the chapter by Faulkner and Bailey, this vol., pp. 1–12, childhood and adolescence are a critical time for bone mineral accrual, and attaining a strong skeleton during growth should help prevent osteoporosis and fractures in later life. Substantial evidence exists that the immature skeleton is more sensitive to mechanical loads than the mature skeleton [1], and thus, it follows that youth is the optimal time in which to initiate an exercise intervention to optimize bone health.

Schools are an ideal medium through which to intervene as they provide the opportunity to reach a large population of children during the majority of the year and throughout the most skeletally responsive years of life. Schools also offer the ability to reach young individuals from across all geographic, ethnic, and socioeconomic strata, and by nature, provide a controlled environment with a captive audience.

This chapter will review the evidence for the effectiveness of school-based interventions for enhancing bone health and discuss important training principles and lessons learned from these intervention trials. It will serve as a guide for educators, administrators, and other pediatric practitioners and health care professionals wishing to implement a school-based osteogenic program in children and adolescents.

Lesson 1: Exercise in Youth Confers Substantial Skeletal Benefit

There have been a number of excellent review papers and chapters in recent years [2–7] which conclude that appropriate physical activity augments bone development. Animal studies suggested that the growing skeleton may be particularly responsive to mechanical loading [1], and several observational studies in humans show that individuals who are the most active during childhood and/or adolescence gain more bone and reached maturity with greater bone mass and strength [6, 8–10].

In addition to the many cross-sectional and prospective observational studies, there are now several school-based physical activity intervention studies which have reported that bone mass and strength can be optimized during growth with relatively modest programs. Overall, these intervention studies (summarized in table 1) used programs that consisted of 3–50 min of physical activity, 2–5 times per week, for 6.5–24 months. The participants consisted of either girls or boys, or mixed groups of boys and girls and ranged in age from 7 to 18 years. A variety of activities were included in the interventions such as jumping, skipping, running, aerobics, and strength training. Further details regarding the interventions are described in table 1.

In all but three of these studies [11–13], a positive benefit of the intervention was observed at the loaded skeletal sites, primarily the hip region (proximal femur) and lumbar spine. The absolute gain in bone mineral in the intervention relative to control groups ranged from 1.2 to 11%, with the greatest changes typically seen at the proximal femur (table 1). These data strongly support the early work conducted in animal studies, which showed that diverse

Table 1. School-based physical activity intervention studies aimed at optimizing bone development

Reference	Subjects and design	Intervention	Results[1]
Prepubertal to early pubertal			
Bradney et al. [34]	Boys Caucasian INT (n = 19); CON (n = 19) Mean age 10.4 ± 0.2 years All TS I 2 schools randomly allocated	*Program:* extra weight-bearing physical activity (basketball, weight training, volleyball, gymnastics, football, aerobics) in addition to regular PE class *Frequency and duration:* 30 min, 3×/week, 8 months *Progression:* none stated *Exercise compliance:* 96%	TB: +1.2% aBMD LS: +2.8% aBMD Femur mid shaft: +5.6% BMC, +5.6% aBMD; NS CSMI and Z
McKay et al. [24]	Girls and boys Asian and Caucasian INT (n = 63); CON (n = 81) Mean age 8.9 ± 0.7 years TS I and II Randomized by school: 5 INT and 5 CON	*Program:* in PE classes, teachers chose activities from a variety of games, circuits, dances which incorporated jumping; 10 tuck jumps performed before PE class, and one time in classroom each week *Frequency and duration:* 10–30 min/session, 3×/week, 8 months *Progression:* as per fitness level of class, more challenging activities added as options after 3 months *Exercise compliance:* not reported	TB: NS LS: NS PF: NS FN: NS GT: +1.2% aBMD

Table 1. (continued)

Reference	Subjects and design	Intervention	Results[1]
Fuchs et al. [31]	Girls and boys Caucasian and Asian INT (n = 45); 44 CON (n = 44) Mean age 7.6 ± 0.2 years All TS I throughout Randomized by classroom to INT or CON within one elementary school	*Program*: intervention took place outside of regular PE classes, supervised by research team; each session: 50–100 2-footed jumps (no box) or drop landings from 61 cm height onto a wooden floor; average GRF of jumps from a 61-cm box was 8.8 ± 0.9 times the body weight *Frequency and duration*: 10 min jumping/session, 3×/week, 7 months *Progression*: week 1–4: progressed from 50 jumps/session (no box), to 80 jumps/session (from a 61-cm-high box); week 5 to end: 100 jumps from box *Exercise compliance*: 96%	LS: +3.1% BMC; +2.0% aBMD FN: +4.5% BMC
MacKelvie et al. [22, 26]	Boys Asian and Caucasian Year 1: INT (n = 61); CON (n = 60) Year 2: INT (n = 31); CON (n = 33) Mean age 10.3 ± 0.6 years TS I throughout Randomized by school (7 INT and 7 CON)	*Program*: classroom-based high-impact jumping program *Frequency and duration*: 10–12 min, 3×/week, 2 school years *Progression*: number of jumps and height of jumps progressed through levels and advanced every 8–10 weeks	Year 1 Year 2 TB: +1.6% BMC NS LS: NS NS PF: +1% aBMD NS FN: NS +4.3% BMC; +7.4% Z

Study	Participants	Intervention	Results
Linden et al. [33] Valdimarsson et al. [36]	Boys and girls Caucasian Boys: INT (n = 81); CON (n = 57); Girls: INT (n = 53); CON (n = 50) 7–9 years old All TS I throughout Not randomized, 4 schools: 1 INT, 3 CON	Year 1: 50 (baseline) to 100 (final) jumps Year 2: 55 jumps (baseline) to 132 (final) jumps *Exercise compliance:* 80% *Program:* physical activity curriculum (60 min/week; increased to 200 min/week); indoor and outdoor activity (ball games, running, jumping, and climbing) *Frequency and duration:* 5×/week, 40-min sessions; 1 school year *Progression:* none	TB: NS LS: +4.7% BMC; +2.8% aBMD FN: –8.4% BMC; –2.6% aBMD (for boys); NS for girls
McKay et al. [28]	Girls and boys Asian and Caucasian INT (n = 51); CON (n = 73) Mean age 10.1 years 65% TS I at baseline Randomized by school	*Program:* Bounce at the Bell – simple jumping program (countermovement jumps); GRFs: 5 times the body weight *Frequency and duration:* 10 jumps, 3×/day, 8 months *Progression:* none *Exercise compliance:* 60%	TB: –1.4% BMC LS: NS PF: +2.1% BMC IT: +2.7% BMC FN: NS
Morris et al. [35]	Girls Ethnicity not stated INT (n = 38); CON (n = 33) Mean age 9.5 ± 0.9 years All premenarcheal (TS I–III; most TS II–III) Not randomized: 2 INT and 2 CON schools	*Program:* one PE teacher supervised intervention program outside of school time; included aerobics, dance, skipping, ball games, weight training *Frequency and duration:* 3×/week, 30 min/session, 10 months (three 10-week school terms, training	TB: +5.5% BMC; +2.3% aBMD LS: +5.5% BMC; +3.6% aBMD; +2.9% vBMD PF: –8.3% BMC; +3.2% aBMD FN: +4.5% BMC; aBMD +10.3%

Table 1. (continued)

Reference	Subjects and design	Intervention	Results[1]
		interrupted for 2 weeks at the end of each term, exercise encouraged over breaks) *Progression*: in 10-week weight training sessions only *Exercise compliance*: 92%	
MacKelvie et al. [21]	Girls Asian and Caucasian INT (n = 32); CON (n = 43) Mean age 10.1 ± 0.5 years All TS I–III at baseline Randomized by school: 7 INT and 7 CON	*Program*: classroom-based high-impact jumping program *Frequency and duration*: 10–12 min, 3×/week, 20 months *Progression*: number of jumps and height of jump progressed through levels and advanced every 8–10 weeks Year 1: 50 (baseline) to 100 (final) jumps Year 2: 55 jumps (baseline) to 132 (final) jumps *Exercise compliance*: not reported	TB: NS LS: +3.7% BMC PF: NS FN: +4.6% BMC
Postmenarcheal Blimkie et al. [11]	Girls Ethnicity not stated INT (n = 16); CON (n = 16) Mean age 16.2 ± 0.2 years All postmenarcheal (TS IV–V) Randomized to INT or CON within 1 school	*Program*: resistance training using hydraulic machines (13 exercises, 4 sets of 10–12 reps); sessions supervised by researchers *Frequency and duration*: session duration not stated, 3×/week, 6.5 months *Progression*: resistance increased every 6 weeks *Exercise compliance*: not reported	TB: NS LS: NS PF: NS

Study	Subjects	Program	Results
Witzke and Snow [12]	Girls Caucasian INT (n = 27); CON (n = 29) Mean age 14.6 ± 0.5 years All postmenarcheal at baseline Not randomized	*Program:* first 3 months: resistance training + plyometrics; final 6 months: plyometrics, including jumps, depth jumps, bounding and hopping on soft surfaces *Frequency and duration:* 30–45 min, 3×/week, 9 months *Progression:* weight training progressed from month 1 to 3: repetitions, sets, and weights gradually increased; plyometric difficulty and number of reps	TB: NS LS: NS PF: NS FN: NS
Nichols et al. [13]	Girls Ethnicity not stated INT (n = 5); CON (n = 11) Mean age 9.5 ± 0.9 years Maturity status not given Randomly assigned to INT or CON	*Program:* 15 resistance exercises; free weights and machines *Frequency and duration:* 30–45 min, 3×/week, 15 months *Progression:* by increasing weight and number of sets *Exercise compliance:* 73%	TB: NS LS: NS PF: NS FN: NS
Across several maturity groups Johannsen et al. [27]	Girls and boys Ethnicity not stated INT (n = 28); CON (n = 26) Age range 3–18 years Randomized by gender and age	*Program:* high-impact jumping program conducted in schools and childcare centers; children jumped off a 45-cm box, 4–5 times the body weight *Frequency and duration:* 25 jumps/day, 5×/week, 12 weeks *Progression:* none stated *Exercise compliance:* 76%	TB: +1% BMC FN: NS Leg: +1.5% BMC Structural measurements: NS

Table 1. (continued)

Reference	Subjects and design	Intervention	Results[1]
Comparison of 2 maturity groups			
Heinonen et al. [19]	Girls Caucasian Premenarcheal: n = 58; TS I–III; INT (n = 25); CON (n = 33); mean age 11.5 ± 1.0 years Postmenarcheal: n = 68; TS II–V; INT (n = 39); CON (n = 33); mean age 13.7 ± 0.9 years Not randomized: schools self-selected to 2 INT; 3 CON	*Program:* jump training sessions, 2- and 1-foot jumps from floor, and on and off a 30-cm box; also did aerobic exercises *Frequency and duration:* 50 min (20 min jumping), 2×/week, 9 months *Progression:* month 1: 100 2-foot jumps, no box; months 7–9: 150 2-foot and 50 1-foot box (30 cm) jumps (multidirectional) *Exercise compliance:* 65%	*Premenarcheal:* LS: +3.3% BMC PF: NS FN: +4.0% BMC Tibial mid shaft: NS *Postmenarcheal:* No significant post-training intergroup differences in any bone parameter
MacKelvie et al. [20] Petit et al. [29]	Girls Asian and Caucasian Prepubertal: n = 70; 44 INT and 26 CON; TS I, mean age 10.1 ± 0.5 years Early pubertal: n = 106; 43 INT and 64 CON; TS II–III, mean age 10.5±0.6 years Randomized by school: 7 INT + 7 CON	*Program:* classroom-based high-impact jumping program *Frequency and duration:* 10–12 min, 3×/week, 7 months *Progression:* number of jumps and height of jump progressed through levels; started with 50 jumps per session and progressed to 100 jumps per session *Exercise compliance:* 80%	*Prepubertal:* NS for any variable *Early pubertal:* TB: NS LS: +1.8% BMC; +1.7% aBMD PF: NS FN: +1.9% BMC; +1.6% aBMD; +3.1% vBMD; +2.3% CSA; +4.0% Z

CON = Control; CSA = bone cross-sectional area; CSMI = cross-sectional moment of inertia; FN = femoral neck; GT = greater trochanter; INT = intervention; IT = intertrochanter; LS = lumbar spine; PF = proximal femur; TB = total body; TS = tanner stage; vBMD = volumetric bone mineral density; Z = section modulus. CSMI and Z are indices of bone bending strength.

[1]Differences are reported as percent difference in change for each bone parameter between intervention and control groups and are all significant at p < 0.05. NS = Not significant.

moderate- to high-impact weight-bearing activities are necessary to optimize bone development. The differences detected between exercise and control groups are likely to be of clinical significance as the greatest benefits were observed at common fracture sites, including the hip and lumbar spine. It has been reported that a 10% decrease in areal bone mineral density (aBMD) represents a 1.5-fold increase in fracture risk. Thus, should these advantages be maintained through adulthood and into senescence, they could help offset the development of skeletal fragility and subsequent fracture. While further details regarding the long-term effects of exercise on bone health are discussed in the chapter by Karlsson, this vol., pp. 121–136, it is evident that more work is needed to confirm a long-term skeletal benefit of these school-based programs.

Lesson 2: Prepuberty and Early Puberty May Provide the Ideal 'Window of Opportunity' in Which to Intervene

Several pieces of evidence led to the idea that prepuberty and early puberty may be an optimal time in which to intervene to optimize skeletal development. First, retrospective human and animal studies clearly indicate that bone responds more favorably to mechanical loading during childhood and adolescence than it does in adulthood [2, 14–16]. In a cross-sectional study comparing differences between the playing and nonplaying arms of young female tennis and squash players, Kannus et al. [17] reported that those individuals who started playing racquet sports before menarche had a 2–4 times greater bone mass in the playing compared to nonplaying arm than those players who started playing after menarche. More recently, a study in pre-, peri- and postpubertal female tennis players reported that the benefits of exercise on bone mass and structural properties (periosteal apposition) occurred during the prepubertal years because the side-to-side differences in favor of the playing arm did not increase with maturity [18]. Although these studies were cross-sectional, they provide a higher level of evidence because by comparing the playing and nonplaying arm of the same person they control for differences in genetics, endocrine status, and nutrition. Together, these data provide strong evidence to suggest that exercise interventions should be commenced before, rather than after menarche (during the prepubertal and early pubertal years).

Several of the school-based interventions support these findings. Interestingly, in the few intervention studies conducted in postmenarcheal girls, exercise failed to augment bone mass relative to controls [11, 12, 19]. Only one study, however, has directly compared the bone response in pre- and postmenarcheal girls within the same study design. Heinonen et al. [19] used the same 9-month step aerobics intervention in both pre- and postmenarcheal girls. In the premenarcheal group, the exercisers gained about 4% more bone mass at the lumbar spine and femoral neck over the 9-month period than controls. In contrast, there were no differences in the change of bone mass for the postmenarcheal girls in the intervention compared to the control group.

While these data support the idea that premenarche is a key time for exercise interventions to optimize bone health in girls, menarche (which occurs around Tanner stage IV[1]) is a relatively late maturational event. To more specifically address the question of 'timing' in the premenarcheal period, MacKelvie et al. [20] conducted a randomized controlled exercise intervention to compare the effectiveness of a progressive loading program performed for 10 min during physical education (PE) classes in premenarcheal girls. One hundred and seventy-seven girls were divided into prepubertal (Tanner stage I) and early pubertal (Tanner stages II and III) groups. Consistent with other studies, the early pubertal girls gained 1.5–3.1% more bone at the femoral neck and lumbar spine than girls of the same maturity status in the control groups. While there was no benefit of the intervention in prepubertal girls over the first year of the intervention [20], all girls in the intervention group gained more bone than controls over 2 years [21]. Interestingly, prepubertal and early pubertal normal-weight (but not overweight) boys had a significant positive response to the same intervention [22], suggesting the 'window of opportunity' may be different for boys and girls. It is also possible that the structural adaptations to exercise are different for boys and girls. However, as discussed in the chapter by Daly, this vol., pp. 33–49, relatively few studies have explored changes in bone geometry or strength following an exercise intervention, and future work is critical to fully address these questions.

Overall, these data suggest that the early pubertal years may represent an optimal time to initiate an exercise program; however, several exercise intervention programs in prepubertal cohorts have also demonstrated a positive skeletal benefit as a result of school-based exercise interventions. Thus, the question as to whether prepuberty or early puberty represents the optimal time to intervene remains unanswered, and it is likely that both maturity stages represent periods of heightened sensitivity to mechanical loading [6, 23].

Lesson 3: Bone Responds to Specific Loading Characteristics

It is well known that bone adapts its structure to its prevailing loads. However, bone may adapt disproportionately to different loading characteristics.

---

[1]Tanner stages are used as a way to evaluate the level of maturity in children. There are five stages based on breast (for girls) and pubic hair (for girls and boys) development that are closely tied to the sex steroid levels in children.

Specifically, the loading modality, intensity, frequency, and duration of the various interventions may have separate effects on bone. Therefore, these factors should be considered when developing an exercise intervention aimed at optimizing bone strength.

Modality

Children participating in weight-bearing activities such as gymnastics and ballet have been shown to have more bone mass than children involved in non-weight-bearing activities such as biking and swimming. Therefore, intervention studies were designed to include weight-bearing activities such as jumping, skipping, plyometrics, resistance training, ball games, and step aerobics. However, many of the exercise interventions involved simultaneous implementation of a variety of these activities, making it difficult to determine which exercise(s) conferred an osteogenic response.

Several interventions included various jumping activities, but only three studies investigated the osteogenic potential of jumping alone. In a study of pre-pubertal children, Fuchs et al. [31] found that children who performed 100 jumps per day, 3 times per week for 7 months had greater gains in femoral neck (+4.5%) and lumbar spine (+3.1%) bone mineral content (BMC) compared to controls. In a randomized study of 28 boys and girls (ages 3–18 years), Johannsen et al. [27] demonstrated that 25 jumps per day, 5 days a week for 12 weeks significantly increased total body and leg BMC (+1, and +1.5%, respectively, $p < 0.05$) compared to controls. In a pilot study of a simple jumping intervention, 'Bounce at the Bell', McKay et al. [28] reported that 10 jumps, 3 times per day were associated with a significant increase in proximal femur (+2.1%, $p < 0.05$) and intertrochanteric (+2.7%) BMC after 8 months. The activities in these interventions were of 'moderate' intensity ranging from 3 to 8 times the body weight [21, 24–28]. Specific details of the intensity level are discussed below.

Similarly, several interventions involved resistance training activities in some capacity; but only two studies utilized resistance training as the sole loading modality. In a randomized study, Blimkie et al. [11] assigned 32 postmenarcheal girls (mean age 16.2 ± 0.2 years) to either 6.5 months of progressive resistance training on hydraulic machines or to a control group. No significant bone changes were demonstrated between groups. Nichols et al. [13] studied the effects of 15 months of resistance exercises, performed 3 times per week for 30–45 min per session in 16-year-old girls (n = 5). Again, no significant between-group differences were demonstrated; but due to the small sample size it is difficult to interpret these findings. Further studies of the skeletal effects of resistance training should be done before this modality is ruled out as osteogenic.

Overall, these studies suggest that weight-bearing impact (jumping) activities, and resistance training all have the potential to be osteogenic. Many of the studies that resulted in favorable skeletal outcomes included various combinations of weight-bearing activities such as running, jumping, and skipping (see table 1 for details). While further studies of the osteogenic capacity of specific physical activities are needed, it can be inferred that a program consisting of a variety of weight-bearing activities with moderate to high impact (discussed below) has the potential to enhance bone health during growth.

Intensity

Exercise is thought to act on the skeleton by generating muscle torque and impact forces, which produce strain, or deformation of bone tissue. Strain is the stimulus, sensed by bone cells, that initiates an adaptive skeletal response. Animal studies have demonstrated that strains that are high in magnitude, rapidly generated, and of abnormal distribution are osteogenic. Therefore, the intensity of a bone-loading exercise intervention can be defined by the ability of the activities to produce these various strain characteristics. It follows that in order to properly characterize the loading intensity, strain magnitude, rate, and distribution must be quantified. However, in vivo strain gauge techniques are invasive, and therefore impractical.

Strain magnitude has been indirectly estimated in several of the skeletal loading interventions by measuring ground reaction forces (GRFs) generated by the various activities. In general, many of the activities included in effective interventions, such as jumping from the ground or a small height, induced GRFs in the range of 3–5 times the body weight [21, 24–28]. In the University of British Columbia Healthy Bones Studies (HBS), activities of this magnitude (3–5 times the body weight) performed for 10 min, 3 times per week were effective at improving bone mass and strength in both boys and girls [20–22, 26, 29]. In another randomized controlled study, children who performed 100 jumps per day off a 61-cm box (associated with a GRF of 8 times the body weight) 3 times per week over 7 months had 3–5% greater gains in bone mass than controls. These studies suggest that osteogenic responses are obtained at loaded skeletal sites using protocols associated with GRFs of 3–8 times the body weight.

While it is difficult to quantify the 'intensity' of bone loading, exercise interventions associated with GRFs of 3–5 times the body weight have been typically classified as being of 'moderate' intensity, whereas those associated with GRFs exceeding 5 times the body weight are considered as being of 'high' intensity. However, it is important to acknowledge that the characteristics of the individual, including type of shoe, landing strategy, height of jump, sex, and stage of maturity, can all influence the peak GRF during any given activity and may contribute to the marked interindividual variability in the osteogenic response to a given loading program. Further work is needed that adequately controls for confounding factors to better quantify the loads for various activities in children. Nonetheless, it is clear that moderate-intensity activities are sufficient to stimulate an adaptive skeletal response during growth.

Strain rate and distribution have not yet been measured in school-based skeletal loading interventions. Nevertheless, it can be inferred that many of the dynamic and multidirectional activities compromising effective loading interventions have produced adequate strain rates and abnormal strain distributions. High strain rates are generated by activities in which the load is rapidly applied or released. This can be accomplished by performing dynamic activities such as jumping, hopping, skipping and by participating in sports incorporating dynamic activities such as volleyball, basketball, and gymnastics. Unusual strain distributions are produced by activities that are novel for that particular person or bone. Activities such as multidirectional jumping, ball sports, dancing, and gymnastics are likely to produce strains in different directions compared to normal physical activities such as walking and running.

Frequency

Frequency can be modified both within the intervention (i.e. the number of jumping repetitions) and by altering the number of times per day or week the intervention is implemented. Animal data show that if activities are high in strain magnitude and of unusual strain distribution, they need not be high in number within a single session. Umemura et al. [30] showed that immature rats which performed 5 jumps per day had similar increases in bone mass and strength compared to those which jumped 40 times per day. Jumping 100 times per day resulted in only slightly greater bone strength gains than 5 jumps per day, suggesting that the immature skeleton does not need to be exposed to a large number of appropriate strains to improve its strength. Frequency of loading has not been well documented in human studies, but school-based interventions involving 100 jumps per day [31], 10 jumps, 3 times per day [28], or 10 min of a variety of jumps [21] resulted in relatively similar and significant gains in bone mass or strength when compared to controls. Overall, these results suggest a threshold response of bone in which relatively few loading cycles per session, of appropriate intensity, are necessary to result in osteogenesis.

Interestingly, a relatively small number of jumps of moderate magnitude may be effective if rest is inserted between sessions [32]. A pilot study of a simple jumping intervention, Bounce at the Bell, showed that 10 jumps, 3 times per day over 8 months was associated with a significant increase in proximal femur (+2.3%) and intertrochanteric (+3.2%) BMC [28]. To perform their jumps, children simply stood next to their desk and jumped for <1 min, 3 times per day when the bell rang. The intervention took less than 3 min per day and required no equipment or special training from teachers. Although more work is needed to confirm these results, these data suggest that interventions can be very simple and short and still be effective at improving bone development.

The optimal number of sessions per week needed to produce a benefit has not been clearly evaluated in humans. The majority of the effective school-based interventions consisted of 2–3 loading sessions per week, with the exception of the Bounce at the Bell [28] and the Swedish Pediatric Osteoporosis Prevention Study [33], which both included 5 sessions per week. As previously mentioned, animal data show that rest inserted between loading bouts increases the sensitivity of bone to subsequent loading, but the ideal amount of time between sessions for humans is not clear and likely depends on the intensity of the activity. From a practical standpoint, many schools in North America only have PE 2–3 times per week (if at all). Positive skeletal benefits demonstrated as a result of interventions implemented only 2–3 times per week indicate that this session frequency is sufficient for enhancing bone health.

Duration

Several of the effective interventions consisted of 30–50 min of weight-bearing physical activity performed 2–5 times per week over a relatively short amount of time (8–12 months) [19, 33–36]. These studies resulted in an average bone mineral advantage of 3% at various skeletal sites. However, similar positive bone gains (approx. 2–3%) were reported in a study involving 10–12 min per day of various jumping and skipping activities, 3 days per week over 7–20 months in both girls [21] and boys [26]. Jumping studies, of only 3 [28] to 10 min [27, 31] in duration, also resulted in comparable bone mineral advantage (approx. 2%) across several skeletal sites. These results indicate that shorter-duration exercise sessions may initiate similar skeletal benefits to those longer in duration. However, even with the same duration of exercise, the type, intensity and frequency of the activity will influence bone's adaptive response and are likely to be more important than the duration. Nonetheless, the studies to date suggest that with the appropriate intensity, 10 min, 3 times per week is an adequate stimulus to improve bone mineral accretion in prepubertal and early pubertal children.

Progression

A final factor to consider when designing a program is the importance of including some type of progression into the program. According to the mechanostat theory, bone must be loaded above what it is typically accustomed to in order to initiate an adaptive response to improve bone mass and strength. Therefore, for loading interventions to be effective, they theoretically should consist of activities which are more intense or diverse than usual activity, and once the skeleton has become accustomed to this new loading environment, interventions must be progressive in order to stimulate further skeletal changes.

In concordance with this theory, the majority of school-based interventions incorporated some form of progression. This was accomplished by increasing the number and/or height of jumps per session; changing the types of activities to make the strains perceived by the bone as 'unusual'; increasing the repetitions, weight lifted, and/or number of sets in resistance training programs, and by removing shoes to increase impact forces. Although it is not clear how quickly bone cells become adapted to any given activity, we recommend incorporating some form of progression at least every 4–8 weeks. It is important to recognize, however, that bone responds to 'unusual' strains, and therefore progression may be as simple as incorporating a new activity or having children jump from side to side instead of up and down. Some examples of how to progress specific activities are included in the sample bone loading program described in the Appendix.

Lesson 4: Calcium Enhances the Effects of Exercise on the Young Skeleton

Three school-based intervention studies have been published that investigated the interactive effects of calcium and exercise on bone health. These studies suggest that there are positive combined effects of exercise and calcium supplementation on the growing skeleton [37–39]. Calcium is considered a threshold nutrient, whereby more than a sufficient amount of calcium will not lead to greater increases in bone mass or strength than adequate levels [40]. Nonetheless, the evidence that calcium may play an important role in augmenting the response of the young skeleton to mechanical loading warrants inclusion of calcium supplementation (preferably through food) in children who are not achieving their adequate intake.

Lesson 5: School-Based Exercise Interventions for Bone Health Are Feasible and Safe

As noted above, many of the successful exercise intervention programs were easily implemented within the existing PE curriculum or in the classroom. The HBS curriculum, for example, consists of 10-min circuits done at the beginning of PE class, 2–3 times per week. On the days children did not have PE, teachers were asked to have children perform 10 tuck jumps (starting from the ground, jumping with knees up to their chest) in their classroom. Activities could be performed with minimal equipment or setup and were simple enough that teachers of any background (e.g. PE, reading, science, math) could implement them. An example of the HBS activities and curriculum is included in the Appendix. There are many different variations to this program, and there are other programs that have also been successful. The HBS sample program is included simply as a guide consisting of different activities known to be osteogenic. Other practical guidelines and activities for both bone and muscle health have recently been published in *Building Strong Bones and Muscles* [41] – or could be as simple as increasing the amount of PE classes per week.

All of the school-based skeletal loading studies proved to be safe as none reported injuries, even with high-impact programs such as jumping from 61-cm boxes (although this was a supervised program involving specialized instructors). Nonetheless, caution should always be used when beginning new activities – for example, children should be taught safe and appropriate landing techniques. It is also important that the programs incorporate the training principle of progressive overload. We recommend starting with body weight-only activities and jumping from the ground, then gradually adding height or diversity to the activities.

Tips to Delivering a Successful School-Based Intervention

Several lessons for a successful school-based intervention to improve bone health can be taken from models for improving general physical activity in children, such as the Action Schools! BC model [42]. Large-scale physical activity intervention studies show that successful interventions are the ones that have commitment from teachers, principals, and children. Involving community partners can help improve support for the project and compliance from children by, for example, donating incentives or prizes to schools that make healthy changes, or by starting programs within the community to encourage more activity or healthy lifestyles outside of the school environment. As many teachers are currently overloaded and not trained specifically to deliver physical activity programs, and because school resources such as money, space and time are limited, programs should be simple and require minimal equipment, space and additional resources. They should be designed so that any teacher could be easily trained to implement them. Developing child-friendly materials and manuals has also been shown to be helpful to improving compliance. Fortunately, many osteogenic activities can be done with minimal equipment or space; require only short-time periods to perform, and activities such as jumping, skipping and hopping are easily implemented by any teacher. Importantly, variety should be included in any program to keep children interested and motivated to participate.

Conclusion

Prospective school-based exercise intervention studies of children that have been conducted for up to 2 years provide convincing evidence to support a central role for exercise in healthy growth and development of the pediatric skeleton. The findings from these studies clearly indicate that mechanical loading dominates bone adaptation during growth, but other factors such as nutrition, disease and hormonal milieu are also likely to mediate the effect. The exact exercise prescription for optimal bone development is not yet clearly defined, but activities that induce moderate impact and produce high strain rates in unusual patterns have a positive effect on bone development, even with only a few loading cycles. Inserting rest between activity bouts also appears to have promise as a means to optimize the bone response to loading. Although prospective, randomized intervention studies are needed to provide definitive answers, there is mounting evidence to suggest that physical activity undertaken in childhood has lasting positive effects on the adult skeleton.

Several important lessons have been learned from the school-based skeletal loading intervention programs in the past decade.

(1) Youth (particularly prepuberty and early puberty) is an important time to implement exercise interventions for the development of a healthy adult skeleton and for the prevention of osteoporosis.

(2) Schools provide an ideal environment in which to intervene on a large-scale population-based level.

(3) Exercise interventions should be progressive and consist of weight-bearing, dynamic, moderately intense, intermittent, and multidirectional activities.

(4) School-based interventions are safe and need not be time-consuming, expensive, or require excessive staff training.

(5) Proper nutrition, particularly adequate calcium intake, is necessary to attain the maximal skeletal benefits of exercise during growth.

Programs that incorporate these guidelines are effective and safe for improving bone mineral accrual in children. It is not clear if this increased bone mass will be maintained until later life for osteoporosis prevention. However, evidence suggests that if activity is maintained at least on some level, so too will the benefits to bone health.

Appendix: Example of Osteogenic Loading Activities, Progressions and a Circuit Program

This is a subset of the activities included in the manual designed by Heather McKay, Kerry MacKelvie-O'Brien, and Moira Petit for the University of British Columbia HBS.

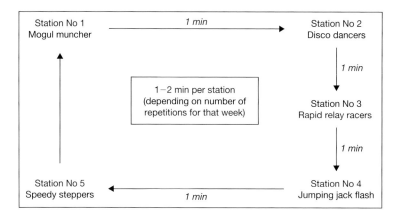

'Healthy Bones' Circuit Training

The activities and program shown below were part of the University of British Columbia's HBS which were reported to successfully enhance bone mineral accrual in young children. The program has been designed to be fun, interactive, fast-paced, time efficient, adaptable and progressive. For optimal skeletal benefits, it is essential that the students complete the 10-min circuit 3 times per week. Stations within the appropriate level can be combined in any way, but due to the progressive nature of the program, stations from different levels should not be combined within one circuit.

Circuit Format

Each circuit is made up of 5 loading stations (your choice) within the appropriate level. It is a good idea to create circuit-travelling teams of 5–6 students per team and then assign teams to a starting station. The students will spend approximately 1–2 min at each station, and rotate on your command (set a time for rotations, i.e., 1 min is recommended to incorporate a rest and time to become familiar with the next station). Prior to starting the circuit, it is important to complete a brief warm-up.

Prior to commencing the program (or new level), explain and demonstrate each station, and monitor correct techniques as laid out in the manual and on posters. Ask students to practice new actions a couple of times before starting the circuit. It is important that the students adopt the proper techniques to ensure safety and avoid injury.

During the first week at a new level, have the students do 10 repetitions at each station (if the jump alternates legs, have them do 10 on each leg), and increase the number of repetitions by 1 each week (for example, week 1: 10 jumps, week 2: 11 jumps, week 3: 12 jumps). When a new level starts, go back to 10 repetitions and increase from there. Color-coded posters can be set up at each station to remind students of the actions. It is also important to have a set direction of movement through the circuit, and you may wish to consider using musical tapes to signal the start and end of each station.

Sample 'Healthy Bones' Circuit Program

Sample 'Healthy Bones' Exercises and Progressions

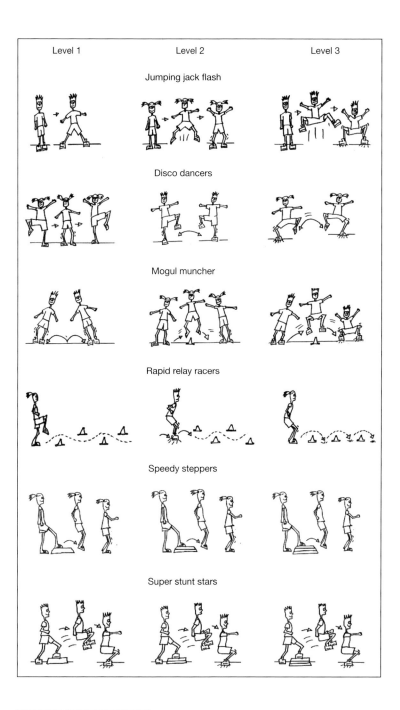

References

1 Forwood M: Mechanical effects on the skeleton: are there clinical implications? Osteoporos Int 2001;12:77–83.
2 Bailey DA, Faulkner RA, McKay HA: Growth, physical activity, and bone mineral acquisition; in Holloszy JO (ed): Exercise and Sport Sciences Reviews. Philadelphia, Lippincott Williams and Wilkins, 1996, pp 233–266.
3 Barr SI, McKay HA: Nutrition, exercise and bone status in youth. Int J Sport Nutr 1998;8: 124–142.
4 McKay HA, Khan KM: Bone mineral acquisition during childhood and adolescence: physical activity as a preventative measure; in Henderson JE, Goltzman D (eds): The Osteoporosis Primer. Cambridge, Cambridge University Press, 2000, pp 170–184.
5 Bass SL, Eser P, Daly R: The effect of exercise and nutrition on the mechanostat. J Musculoskelet Neuronal Interact 2005;5:239–254.
6 MacKelvie KJ, Khan KM, McKay HA: Is there a critical period for bone response to weight-bearing exercise in children and adolescents? A systematic review. Br J Sports Med 2002;36: 250–257.
7 Hind K, Burrows M: Weight-bearing exercise and bone mineral accrual in children and adolescents: a review of controlled trials. Bone 2007;40:14–27.
8 Bailey DA, McKay HA, Mirwald RL, Crocker PRE, Faulkner RA: A six-year longitudinal study of the relationship of physical activity to bone mineral accrual in growing children: the University of Saskatchewan bone mineral accrual study. J Bone Miner Res 1999;14:1672–1679.
9 Petit MA, Beck TJ, Lin HM, Bentley C, Legro RS, Lloyd T: Femoral bone structural geometry adapts to mechanical loading and is influenced by sex steroids: the Penn State Young Women's Health Study. Bone 2004;35:750–759.
10 Bass SL: The prepubertal years: a uniquely opportune stage of growth when the skeleton is most responsive to exercise? Sports Med 2000;30:73–78.
11 Blimkie C, Rice S, Webber C: Effects of resistance training on bone mineral content and density in adolescent females. Can J Physiol Pharmacol 1996;74:1025–1033.
12 Witzke KA, Snow CM: Effects of plyometric jump training on bone mass in adolescent girls. Med Sci Sport Exerc 2000;32:1051–1057.
13 Nichols DL, Sanborn CF, Love AM: Resistance training and bone mineral density in adolescent females. J Pediatr 2001;139:494–500.
14 Bailey D, McCulloch R: Osteoporosis: are there childhood antecedents for an adult health problem? Can J Pediatr 1992;4:130–134.
15 Parfitt AM: The two faces of growth: benefits and risks to bone integrity. Osteoporos Int 1994;4: 382–398.
16 Forwood MR, Burr DB: Physical activity and bone mass: exercises in futility? Bone Miner 1993;21:89–112.
17 Kannus P, Haapasalo H, Sankelo M, Sievanen H, Pasanen M, Heinonen A, Oja P, Vuori I: Effect of starting age of physical activity on bone mass in the dominant arm of tennis and squash players. Ann Intern Med 1995;123:27–31.
18 Bass SL, Saxon L, Daly RM, Turner CH, Robling AG, Seeman E, Stuckey S: The effect of mechanical loading on the size and shape of bone in pre-, peri-, and postpubertal girls: a study in tennis players. J Bone Miner Res 2002;17:2274–2280.
19 Heinonen A, Sievanen H, Kannus P, Oja P, Pasanen M, Vuori I: High-impact exercise and bones of growing girls: a 9-month controlled trial. Osteoporos Int 2000;11:1010–1017.
20 MacKelvie KJ, McKay HA, Khan KM, Crocker PRE: Defining the window of opportunity: a school-based loading intervention augments bone mineral accrual in early, but not pre-, pubertal girls. J Pediatr 2001;139:501–508.
21 MacKelvie KJ, Khan KM, Petit MA, Crocker PRE, McKay HA: A school-based exercise intervention elicits substantial bone health benefits: a 2-year randomized controlled trial in girls. Pediatrics 2003;112:e447.

22   MacKelvie KJ, McKay HA, Petit MA, Moran O, Khan KM: Bone mineral response to a 7-month randomized controlled, school-based jumping intervention in 121 prepubertal boys: associations with ethnicity and body mass index. J Bone Miner Res 2002;17:834–844.

23   Bass S, Pearce G, Bradney M, Hendrich E, Delmas PD, Hardy A, Seeman E: Exercise before puberty may confer residual benefits in bone density in adulthood: studies in active prepubertal and retired female gymnasts. J Bone Miner Res 1998;13:500–507.

24   McKay HA, Petit MA, Schutz RW, Prior JC, Barr SI, Khan KM: Augmented trochanteric bone mineral density after modified physical education classes: a randomized school-based exercise intervention study in prepubescent and early pubescent children. J Pediatr 2000;136: 156–162.

25   McKay HA, Tsang G, Heinonen A, MacKelvie K, Sanderson D, Khan KM: Ground reaction forces associated with an effective elementary school based jumping intervention. Br J Sports Med 2004;39:10–14.

26   MacKelvie KJ, Petit MA, Khan KM, Beck TJ, McKay HA: Bone mass and structure are enhanced following a 2-year randomized controlled trial of exercise in prepubertal boys. Bone 2004;34: 755–764.

27   Johannsen N, Binkley T, Englert V, Neiderauer G, Specker B: Bone response to jumping is site-specific in children: a randomized trial. Bone 2003;33:533–539.

28   McKay HA, MacLean L, Petit M, MacKelvie-O'Brien K, Janssen P, Beck T, Khan KM: 'Bounce at the Bell': a novel program of short bouts of exercise improves proximal femur bone mass in early pubertal children. Br J Sports Med 2005;39:521–526.

29   Petit MA, McKay HA, MacKelvie KJ, Heinonen A, Khan KM, Beck TJ: A randomized school-based jumping intervention confers site and maturity-specific benefits on bone structural properties in girls: a hip structural analysis study. J Bone Miner Res 2002;17:363–372.

30   Umemura Y, Ishiko T, Yamauchi T, Kurono M, Mashiko S: Five jumps per day increase bone mass and breaking force in rats. J Bone Miner Res 1997;12:1480–1485.

31   Fuchs RK, Bauer JJ, Snow CM: Jumping improves hip and lumbar spine bone mass in prepubescent children: a randomized controlled trial. J Bone Miner Res 2001;16:148–156.

32   Robling AG, Burr DB, Turner CH: Recovery periods restore mechanosensitivity to dynamically loaded bone. J Exp Biol 2001;204:3389–3399.

33   Linden C, Ahlborg H, Gardsell P, Valdimarsson O, Stenevi-Lundgren S, Besjakov J, Karlsson MK: Exercise, bone mass and bone size in prepubertal boys: one-year data from the pediatric osteoporosis prevention study. Scand J Med Sci Sports 2006, E-pub ahead of print.

34   Bradney M, Pearce G, Naughton G, Sullivan C, Bass S, Beck T, Carlson J, Seeman E: Moderate exercise during growth in prepubertal boys: changes in bone mass, size, volumetric density, and bone strength: a controlled prospective study. J Bone Miner Res 1998;13:1814–1821.

35   Morris FL, Naughton GA, Gibbs JL, Carlson JS, Wark JD: Prospective 10-month exercise intervention in premenarcheal girls: positive effects on bone and lean mass. J Bone Miner Res 1997;12: 1453–1462.

36   Valdimarsson O, Linden C, Johnell O, Gardsell P, Karlsson MK: Daily physical education in the school curriculum in prepubertal girls during 1 year is followed by an increase in bone mineral accrual and bone width – data from the prospective controlled Malmo pediatric osteoporosis prevention study. Calcif Tissue Int 2006;78:65–71.

37   Iuliano-Burns S, Saxon L, Naughton G, Gibbons K, Bass SL: Regional specificity of exercise and calcium during skeletal growth in girls: a randomized controlled trial. J Bone Miner Res 2003;18: 156–162.

38   Stear SJ, Prentice A, Jones SC, Cole J: Effect of a calcium and exercise intervention on the bone mineral status of 16- to 18-year-old adolescent girls. Am J Clin Nutr 2003;77:985–992.

39   Specker B, Binkley T: Randomized trial of physical activity and calcium supplementation on bone mineral content in 3- to 5-year-old children. J Bone Miner Res 2003;18:885–892.

40   Heaney RP, Abrams S, Dawson-Hughes B, Looker A, Marcus R, Matkovic V, Weaver C: Peak bone mass. Osteoporos Int 2000;11:985–1009.

41 Fishburne GJ, McKay HA, Berg SP: Building Strong Bones and Muscles. Champaign, Human Kinetics, 2006.

42 Naylor PJ, Macdonald HM, Zebedee JA, Reed KE, McKay HA: Lessons learned from Action Schools! BC – an 'active school' model to promote physical activity in elementary schools. J Sci Med Sport 2006;9:413–423.

Moira Petit, PhD
University of Minnesota
School of Kinesiology
110 Cooke Hall
Minneapolis, MN 55455 (USA)
Tel. +1 612 625 5506, Fax +1 612 625 9380
E-Mail mpetit@umn.edu

Subject Index

Distance runners
  bone turnover in nutritional amenorrhea
    86, 87
  effects on bone geometry and strength
    during growth 36
Dual-energy X-ray absorptiometry (DXA)
  bone strength assessment 17, 18
  fracture risk analysis 3–5
  quantitative computed tomography
    comparison 34
  school-based exercise intervention trials
    42–45

Energy
  deprivation
    fracture risk during growth 111
    menstrual cycle disturbance 83, 92,
      93, 97
  nutrition-exercise interaction in bone
    health during growth 59, 60
Estrogen
  bone growth regulation 28, 38
  receptor polymorphisms 68, 72
Exercise
  bone mineral acquisition effects 7
  developmental exercise and fracture
    prevention in later life
    athlete studies 130–133
    bone mass and structure response 123,
      124
    duration of effects after detraining
      bone mass 124–128
      bone mineral density 124
      bone structure 128, 129
    study design 122, 123, 129, 130
  effects on bone geometry and strength
    during growth
    high-impact athletic training 35–40
    overview 35
    recreational and leisure activity
      40, 41
    school-based intervention, see School-
      based exercise intervention trials
  gene-environment interaction during
    growth 69–74
  male athletes and intense training effects
    on endocrine function 95, 96

menstrual cycle disturbance, see
  Menstrual cycle disturbance
nutrition interaction in bone health during
  growth
  calcium 53–57
  concept of interaction 51–53
  energy 59, 60
  protein 59, 60
  vitamin D 58

Fractures
  bone mineral density in risk analysis 3, 4
  epidemiology during growth
    fracture patterns 103, 104
    overview 102, 103
    rate variation with age and sex 104
    repeated fractures 104, 105
    risk factors
      bone mineral density 107, 108
      first fracture 106, 107
      genetics 109, 110
      intrauterine factors 110
      medications 109
      musculoskeletal weakness 108
      nutrition 110–112
      obesity 108, 109
      smoking 112
    trauma 105
    trends 105
  genetics 7, 8
  management during growth 114, 115
  osteoporosis
    consequences 2
    economic impact 2, 3
    risks 2, 121, 122
  peak bone mass effects in later life 66
  prevention during growth
    environment safety 112
    general strategies 113–115
    limiting risk taking behavior 114
    management of low bone mineral
      density 113

Genetics
  bone mass and strength 67–69
  environment interactions in bone growth
    69–74

fracture risk 7, 8, 109, 110
Ground reaction force (GRF), bone
 response in school-based exercise
 intervention 148
Growth hormone (GH)
 bone mineral acquisition effects 6
 menstrual cycle disturbance levels 83,
  92, 93
Gymnastics, effects on bone geometry and
 strength during growth 36, 123

High-impact athletic training, effects on
 bone geometry and strength during
 growth 35–40

Insulin-like growth factor-I (IGF-I)
 binding proteins 93
 bone growth regulation 28, 29
 male athletes and intense training effects
  95, 96
 menstrual cycle disturbance levels 83,
  92–94
 protein and energy nutrition effects on
  levels 59–61
 therapy, bone formation 97

Leptin
 menstrual cycle disturbance levels
  92, 95
 osteotrophic effects 94, 95
Low birth weight, fracture risk during
 growth 110
Low-density lipoprotein receptor-related
 protein 5 (LRP5)
 polymorphisms and bone health 68, 69
 sclerostin antagonism 72

Menstrual cycle disturbance (MCD)
 bone turnover in nutritional amenorrhea
  85–92
 endocrine changes 83
 energy deprivation role 83
 etiology 81, 82
 features 82, 83
 insulin-like growth factor-I levels 83,
  92–94
 leptin levels 92, 95

recommendations for prevention and
 treatment 96, 97
skeletal parameters 83–85
Milk, avoidance and fracture risk during
 growth 111, 112

Nutrition, *see also* specific nutrients
 bone mineral acquisition effects 6, 7
 bone turnover in nutritional amenorrhea
  85–88
 exercise interaction in bone health during
  growth
  calcium 53–57
  concept of interaction 51–53
  energy 59, 60
  protein 59, 60
  vitamin D 58
 fracture risk during growth 110–112
 gene-environment interactions during
  growth 69–74

Obesity, fracture risk during growth 108,
 109
Osteocalcin, anorexia nervosa levels 88
Osteoporosis
 back strength training and compression
  fracture prevention in postmenopausal
  women 132
 fracture
  consequences 2
  economic impact 2, 3
  risks 2, 121, 122
 genetics 69
 juvenile disease 6
 prevalence 1, 2, 34, 137

Peak bone mass
 attainment 3
 factors affecting bone mineral acquisition
  6–8
 prediction of bone mineral status in older
  adults 4, 65–67
Physical education, *see* School-based
 exercise intervention trials
Protein, nutrition-exercise interaction in
 bone health during growth 59, 60